When Christians Say, "I Believe Life Starts at Conception"

Christopher W. Bogosh

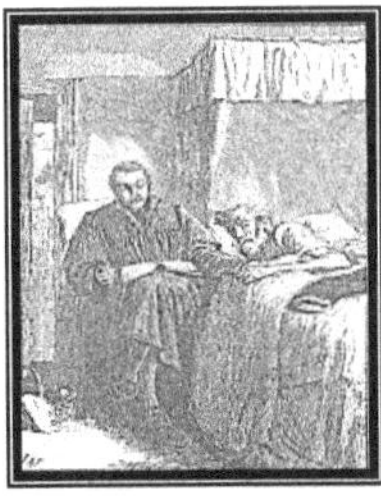

Good Samaritan Books

To my sister in Christ, Dr. Heidi Klessig:
fellow laborer in God's vineyard and
compassionate pro-life advocate.

Contents

Foreword: Heidi Klessig, MD
Retired Anesthesiologist
Pain Management Specialist

When Christians Say, "I Believe Life Starts at Conception" is a book about life and death. As living souls created in the image of God, humans experience life as a body-soul unity. We ask questions like "Who am I? What is my story? What is life about? How can I know what is true, and to whom am I accountable?"

At the same time, our physical bodies require our attention. We need air, food, water, and warmth. As long as our souls are combined with our physical bodies, all body systems work together in amazing harmony. Even as we sleep, our hearts keep beating, and our lungs continue breathing. Illness or an injury may disrupt the comfort and flow of our lives, but thanks to our wonderful healing potential combined with holistic and modern medicine, many now live with conditions once thought incurable. But because we are mortal, eventually, our souls depart to return to the Lord who gave them, and our bodies lose the ability to function as an integrated whole and become corpses.

Christians are familiar with the idea that life begins at conception. But because the age in which we live is predominantly humanistic and utilitarian, our definitions of death have become more elastic. In 1968, doctors at Harvard Medical School redefined death to include people in an "irreversible" coma. There were no new studies, tests, or evidence that people in a coma are dead. Comatose people have beating hearts and breathing lungs, and their body systems still work together in an integrated fashion: they are still biologically very much alive. However, because doctors had found that only organs from living donors could be successfully transplanted, they redefined death to skirt the ethical and legal culpability of murdering incapacitated people for their organs.

While this redefinition of death is hotly debated amongst physicians, lawyers, and bioethicists, the public has been kept in the dark. This book intends to change that. Some of the facts in this book may surprise you, but they're medically accurate. During my medical training, I provided anesthesia for an organ donor and saw firsthand how he responded to incisions and surgery. I have no doubt now that his life-giving spirit was still in union with his body—he was still alive—even though he was declared dead.

You may wonder how the medical establishment could have gone so wrong for so long since it's been over fifty years since the definition of death was changed. It's helpful to remember that medicine has a long history of having to correct itself. When Dr. Ignaz Semmelweis proposed in 1847 that doctors wash their hands before treating patients, his (correct) idea was met with such scorn and derision that he suffered a nervous breakdown and died in a mental institution. This is just one example of hundreds mentioned in history books on the development of medical science. Only with constant questioning and correcting can medicine improve patient outcomes.

But this is not just a medical book. *When Christians Say, "I Believe Life Starts at Conception"* also addresses the faulty worldview that drives so many physicians, bioethicists, and clergy. Many today see living human beings made in the image of God as just "molecules in motion," or they define disabled people lacking mental abilities as being unworthy of life.

With his background in nursing and theology and his experience as an author, Christopher W. Bogosh has a unique ability to explain the Christian view of life, death, and medical care. He is committed to 2 Corinthians 10:5, "Casting down arguments and every high thing that exalts itself against the knowledge of God, bringing every thought into captivity to the obedience of Christ." In this book, Bogosh uses the Word of God to define the meaning of life and death, and then he successfully applies this knowledge to medical science. He uses a holistic approach in the best sense of the word: his prescription addresses the needs of our bodies and the questions of our souls.

Christians desire to love and honor God with all their heart, mind, soul, and strength. The insights found in *When Christians Say, "I Believe Life Starts at Conception"* will help us honor God (and those in vulnerable conditions made in His image) with our medical decision-making.

Preface

Life is a narrative built on history and rooted in guiding authorities—it's a story. All stories have universal and transcendent symbols, or archetypes, that connect the elements of the historical narrative to the story of a person's present life. Medical doctors, philosophers, theologians, and politicians are some of today's authorities controlling life's stories. They are also characters in the historical narrative of life, however, believing in the stories they view as authoritative.

I, too, am guided by authorities. Therefore, I'll be looking to the expertise of others to support the overarching narrative of this book and its application to our current setting. Nevertheless, my plotline is straightforward: if Christians believe human life starts after a sperm fertilizes an egg (conception), then it cannot end until cardiopulmonary cessation and bodily disintegration occurs (natural death). I set these biological facts of science into the context of Holy Scripture and explain how this needs to guide the Christian's approach to modern medicine in the story of life today.

When Christians Say, "I Believe Life Starts at Conception" is the result of reflecting on this subject for many years. As a result, I owe a debt of gratitude to several people, too numerous to mention. Please accept a general thank you, I don't want to be verbose. Also, please know that when you come to mind, I do not hesitate to pray for each of you.

For this book, however, two people deserve special thanks. Doctor Heidi Klessig, to whom this book is dedicated, and Robin Bogosh, to whom I dedicated my life. I can't express enough thanks for these two sisters in the LORD.

First, after a fantastic work of God's providence a few years ago, Dr. Klessig and I became acquainted (see *Harvesting Organs & Cherishing Life*). Thanks to her expertise as a Doctor of Medicine and anesthesiologist, the things I've been writing about for over a decade have received greater credibility. For me, she placed her expert medical stamp on conclusions I made as a registered nurse practicing at the bedside and emboldened me as a writer of Christian medical ethics. The effect of her ministry on me was greater clarity and zeal.

Second, only in chronological succession to my dear sister Heidi is my wife, Robin. She, too, is a registered nurse. Most of Robin's nursing career was practiced with great success at the managerial and director levels. Her professional life, however, pales in comparison as God's gift to me as a godly wife, and my best friend in our life story. Once again, like those mentioned above, an entire book could be written to express my gratitude for all she has done. For this book, however, I would like to focus on one creative act of genius — the excellent book cover.

Christopher W. Bogosh
Season of Christmas

Introduction

I have a shameful secret, those close to me know about it, but others don't. When I was a teenager, I was involved in an intimate relationship that resulted in a pregnancy. My girlfriend's mother made her get an abortion, and I had to pay for half of it. The abortion didn't matter much to me at the time. Sadly, I was more concerned about the expense! Suffice it to say, I was not always pro-life or a sincere Christian.

I received the sacrament of baptism as an infant. Still, the way I lived as a young adult was completely unlike Jesus. My philosophy about life was rooted in hedonism, moral relativism, and narcissism. It wasn't until my twenty-sixth birthday that I became a genuine Christian. The grace of baptism came to life that year, and I experienced true joy, peace, and eternal life for the first time.

There was a noticeable change in 1994. The old Chris was crucified with Christ, and the new Chris came to life. By the work of the Holy Spirit, I experienced repentance, and with sorrow for my ungodly living, I turned to the Creator of life with a desire to do his will. That same year, I also realized that many people don't like it when Christians share their new-found beliefs.

During my maternity rotation in nursing school, my instructor assigned me a woman whose baby died shortly after birth. The mother knew the unborn child had congenital abnormalities and was offered an abortion during the pregnancy. However, she and her husband decided against the abortion and went forward with having the baby. According to the parents after the birth of the child, with obvious visible deformities, many tears were shed. They didn't regret their decision, however, and the opportunity to see, hold, and comfort their infant boy until he passed from life to death. During our post-clinical roundtable, I had to present the case to the group.

I still remember sitting at the brown table with the black plastic border. Bright lights were beaming down on us, and the eyes of nine females were staring at me—the only male. I presented the sad situation, and the instructor asked me: "Do you think she should've had the abortion?" My past flashed before my mind, and I gulped. Feeling ashamed for the lack of concern for my unborn baby in the past and convicted, I meekly muttered, "No."

I didn't know why I said no at the time, but I *felt* like having an abortion was wrong. Seven of my fellow students looked away from me, breathed out heavily, and became agitated. One, however, stared at me and smiled. Then the discussion was about why the mother should have had the abortion until the smiling colleague said: "My mother was faced with a choice to abort me. I'm glad she didn't." The room fell silent after that, and the instructor moved on to another colleague's presentation of the happy birth of a healthy baby.

Today, I know why I felt that way, but back then, I didn't. According to Holy Scripture, the "old heart" of stone was taken away. My belief about life was no longer "to each their own," and moral relativism was exposed. At the same time, I received a "new heart" with God's Law written on it by the Holy Spirit (Ezek. 36:25–27; John 3). "You shall not murder" applies to un-formed and unborn babies in the womb (Ps. 139:13; Exod. 20:13). Less than a decade had passed since that tragic teenage episode, and now my pro-life campaign was set into motion during nursing school.

After I received my nursing degree and be-came licensed to practice, I enrolled in seminary and started to train for pastoral ministry. Some-how, however, it seemed the more I was taught theology and its application to medical science, the less I trusted the feeling I had in that brightly illuminated conference room. A perplexing phe-nomenon, to say the least. Faith should deepen as we learn about God's will and its application to life, not lessen. I was learning about excep-tions to the rule and new approaches to medical ethics, many of which I question today.

Although I never returned to the maternity ward as a nurse or pastor, I've cared profession-ally for thousands of people. I've ministered to those with aggressive cancers and chronic ill-nesses who were racked by pain, worry, suffering, and regret. I've been at the bedside of those in the throes of death, gasping for their final breaths. I've cared for those losing themselves and others due to dementia. I gazed in disbelief at a child with hydrocephalus, whose enormous head dwarfed his little body. I've cared for several children with cystic fibrosis, those in a persistent vegetative state (PVS), and others with severe mental impairment due to genetic defects or accidents. I would be remiss, not to mention the hundreds of unresponsive people with a beating heart on a ventilator. I thought a lot about the futility of aggressive treatments, what it means to be a human being, and my responsibility to my sick neighbors as a Christian.

Throughout the years, I've also heard many answers for people struggling with the above-mentioned conditions. Most of them reflected the reason for the abortion my colleagues gave during nursing school, which had to do with eliminating a burden and serving the selfish desires of others. Here are some of the solutions:

- We should not just allow abortion as a choice but require it for unborn babies with congenital abnormalities.

- We should mandate organ donation for people declared brain dead with viable organs to transplant.
- We should legalize physician-assisted suicide in all fifty states.
- We should legalize active euthanasia for people with mental impairment, and terminal illnesses.

These answers do not value life, and they should raise the ire of anyone claiming to be pro-life, but truth be told, some Christians are complicit in similar ways.

After the leak of Justice Alito's draft decision to overturn Roe v. Wade in May of 2022, my local newspaper, *News Leader*, solicited editorials. What I wrote for the paper will help to flesh out my point further and emphasize the thrust behind *When Christians Say, "I Believe Life Starts at Conception."*

> "The Abortion Issue & Integrity"
> Of all the institutions in the federal government, one would expect integrity to reign in the U.S. Supreme Court. Sadly, this is no longer the case due to a leaker, a government employee lacking integrity. In fact, I'm convinced that the whole issue related to abortion is rife with integrity problems, not only among those who advocate Roe v. Wade but

also among those who oppose it.

Integrity is the quality of being honest, which means accepting what is true to be reality. It is an indisputable fact of human development that if a sperm penetrates an egg in a womb, a unique person will develop and be born. Of course, that's if all goes as expected. Second, integrity has the quality of being moral and ethical. Herein lies the rub in the United States. People cannot agree on what's moral and ethical.

Pro-life people are fond of saying, "Life starts at conception!" Personally, I'm convinced that this is true. This position, however, calls into question other practices permitted under U.S. law, such as abortion, that I cannot accept, at least if I want to maintain my integrity. For example, the Uniform Determination of Death Act (UDDA) permits harvesting organs from people declared brain dead who still have a beating heart. If I hold that life starts at conception, then this is at least five weeks before the brain develops. For this reason, I see the UDDA the same way I view Roe v. Wade. As a result, I'm not a registered organ donor, nor do I assume medical practices are always moral and ethical if they are legal.

In fact, many pro-life people would be shocked at the medical research, procedures, and products permitted under U.S. law that violate pro-life convictions, especially those that use human tissues collected in different stages of development after pro-choice abortions. The COVID-19 vaccines are an example. While it's easy to carry an antiabortion sign and declare, "Life begins at conception," living this conviction out is not always straightforward. Nor is it easy for a pregnant teen who is afraid and may have been exploited.

Rape and incest are wicked. Sometimes these heinous acts result in a pregnancy. Sexually active lifestyles leading to unwanted pregnancies are real issues, not to mention pregnancies that may put the mother's life at risk or the challenging commitment to a child born with genetic defects. These are not easy problems to navigate, and they are highly complex. Make no mistake. Nevertheless, every moral and ethical solution to them is rooted in guiding authorities or beliefs.

Still, integrity requires being honest with reality. As I said above: "It is an indisputable fact of human development that if a sperm penetrates an egg in a womb, a unique person will develop and be born." This is a cellular form of a human that needs life support from a selfless mother—like those we honored this past Mother's Day.

Pro-choice advocates argue, "My body, my choice!" President Biden was correct when he said this is a choice to "abort a child." Let that Freudian slip sink in. Biden also said, "I'm a child of God; I exist," and based our human rights on this belief. According to Biden's conviction, human rights are rooted in the fact that we exist because we

> are the offspring of God. This should mean that God has the ultimate right to begin, end, and direct what we do with life, not us.
>
> Thus, his children will honor human life from conception to natural death and seek to cherish it with integrity in between.

In my experience, I've encountered many Christians who condemn abortion, don't think twice about receiving COVID-19 vaccines manufactured from aborted babies, and receive organs from unresponsive people declared dead with objective signs of life. Most Christians are unaware of their inconsistencies, but some are, and they will even try to defend their positions.

This brings me back to my original point, "Somehow, however, it seemed, the more I was taught about theology and its application to medical science, the less I trusted the feeling I had in that brightly illuminated conference room." I'm not suggesting Christians should be anti-intellectual. On the contrary, they need to think more critically about modern medicine and be willing to re-evaluate the traditions they've come to embrace, especially those who counsel other Christians about the matters I mentioned. These inconsistencies do not stem from medical science or Holy Scripture. They originate from affirming views of what it means to be human, developed by theologians locked by time into a specific historical space.

Historically, Christian theologians have gravitated toward Plato or Aristotle to define human life or the image of God in human beings. Aside from not being biblical, the major problem is the philosophies of Plato and Aristotle, which are ultimately reduced to various forms of dualism, may permit a belief that a fertilized egg is a human life in potential, a non-responsive person with a beating heart dependent on life support may be defined as dead, and a person without mental capacity may no longer be viewed as possessing personhood. This last point developed in earnest during the Middle Ages, and it essentially taught that the image of God was seen in the soul's faculties of reason, will, and virtue.

It didn't matter much until the middle of the twentieth century if a cluster of intellectual or moral attributes defined what it meant to be a human being. Most people before the 1960s were not unresponsive with beating hearts, but if they were, I can assure you they would be viewed as living—probably as sleeping. As medicine developed in the sixteenth century, the physician Andreas Vesalius was convicted of murder for cutting a comatose person open with a beating heart.

It wasn't until 1968 after Dr. Henry Beecher published an article that appeared in the *Journal of the American Medical Association*, "A Definition of Irreversible Coma: Report of the Ad Hoc Committee of the Harvard Medical School to Examine the Definition of Brain Death," that a new definition of death would emerge. Among other reasons, Beecher wrote the article to prevent the prosecution of physicians who wanted to declare unresponsive people dead with objective signs of life for legal, economic, and exploitative reasons. This article laid the groundwork for the Uniform Determination of Death Act (UDDA) in 1981, which permits a legal definition of death for unresponsive organ donors with objective signs of life.

According to Holy Scripture, what makes us human is much more fundamental than reason, will, and virtue. Humans possess a unique form of life. This is the primary teaching of Genesis 2:7, "the LORD God formed the man from the dust of the ground and breathed into his nostrils the breath of life, and the man became a living being." Humans are "ground" and "breath of life" beings. It is this fundamental union of "breath of life" or "spirit," as the Hebrew word may be translated, from the Creator united to material creation that makes a "living being" or "living soul" (KJV) an image bearer of the Creator of life, nothing more.

The writer of Genesis wrote earlier about humanity in general, "God created man in his image, in the image of God he created him; male and female he created them" (Gen. 1:27). This was after the Creator made all the living creatures "according to their kinds" and declared his intention to create humans (vv. 24–25). The Creator is the fountain of all life, but there is a difference between human life and other biological life forms. Humans bear the image of the Creator as mortal beings with unique male and female identities, and they are different from other living creatures. Both women and men are invested with the authority to care for the creation, and they are to procreate to fill the world with other unique material creations and God-breathed beings (vv. 26, 28).

Genesis provides three strands of timeless truths to inform Christian anthropology.

1. The spirit from the Creator, in union with the material creation, creates a living human being to bear his image.
2. The Creator of life is the fountain of all life, but there is a difference between human life and other forms of life. Humans bear the image of the Creator as mortal beings with unique male and female identities.
3. Men and women are invested with authority to care for the creation, which includes cherishing human life, and to procreate to make fellow image bearers of the Creator to fill the world.

According to Holy Scripture, this is what it means to be a human being created in the image of God.

Most importantly, for Christians confronted by modern medical advances, this has nothing to do with possessing intellectual, moral, or volitional attributes. Still, it has everything to do with having biological signs of human life in-

side the womb and outside of it in the Creator's world to serve the Creator.

Jesus affirmed this teaching in the Gospels, and Paul did in his Epistles. "He is not the God of the dead, but of the living, for to him all are alive," Jesus said (Luke 20:38). He goes on in Mark's Gospel, "at the beginning of creation God 'made them male and female'" and talked about marriage and procreation to fill the world with image bearers of the Creator (10:6).

In Paul's speech to the philosophers in Athens, he said:

> 'For in him we live and move and have our being.' As some of your own poets have said, 'We are his offspring.' Therefore since we are God's offspring, we should not think that the divine being is like gold or silver or stone — an image made by man's design and skill" (Acts 17:28–29).

On the contrary, Paul says elsewhere the Creator creates men and women to declare his image in the creation as his achievement and to declare his existence (cf. Col. 3:10). It's not the other way around.

There is another thread weaved through this

biblical teaching about Christian anthropology, one that cuts us down to size: humans are dependent beings. People reflect the Creator's image, but they are not God. Everyone depends on the creation and the Creator for ongoing life, just like a fertilized egg in a womb or a "brain-dead" organ donor with a beating heart on a ventilator. Of course, unborn babies and unresponsive people don't appear conscious or have moral volition; nevertheless, they still have God's breath of life and bear the Creator's image. At this vulnerable time, they are more dependent and require fellow image-bearers who share their mortality to show them love, mercy, and compassion.

In the following chapters, we will start with an overview of today's definition of death and its non-scientific assumptions rooted in materialism/monism, which assumes only matter and energy exist and the deterministic natural laws that govern them. Then we will journey back into the ancient world to consider the Old Testament view of what it means to be a human being created in the image of God and how that informs the Christian today.

Moving on into chapter two, we will consider

the unique human beings the Creator created people to be, along with the Creator's purpose in the world he created. We will look at Jesus, the Lamb of God/Second Adam. In chapter three, we will consider dualism in Holy Scripture by focusing on Paul, and then we will look at some of its dangers for Christians who appeal to Greek philosophy to define Christian anthropology. The last chapter shows how modern judgments about human life in the United States (US) are like those that were espoused in Nazi Germany.

1

Dependent God-Breathed Dust

You may be surprised to find out that the biological sciences do not support today's definition of death in the United States (US). A legal fiction (not true to the facts but permissible by law) rooted in materialism (i.e., only matter/energy exist and the natural laws that govern them) and a worldview (e.g., atheism, pantheism, or deism) at odds with Christianity does.

As noted in the Introduction, death was redefined in 1981, and this definition was codified as federal law in the Uniform Determination of Death Act (UDDA). The UDDA states:

An individual who has sustained either (1) ir-

reversible cessation of circulatory and respiratory functions, or (2) irreversible cessation of
all functions of the entire brain, including the
brain stem, is dead. A determination of death
must be made in accordance with accepted
medical standards.

Since the UDDA became US law, it has been controversial because of its non-scientific assumptions. Presently, the Uniform Law Commission
(ULC) is working on updates to the UDDA.

In the 2008 affirmation of the UDDA, *Contro-
versies in the Determination of Death: A White Paper
by the President's Council on Bioethics*, the Chairman had to write a statement opposing the ma-
jority consensus that supported the ongoing application of the UDDA as US law. In the "Personal Statement of Edmund D. Pellegrino,
M.D.," he writes the following:

> The Chairman's first obligation concerning
> any Council report is to ensure that it fairly
> and accurately reflects the opinions of the
> Council members and that the evidence and
> research supporting those opinions is com-
> plete and reliably presented. …Like any
> Council member, the Chairman is free to ex-
> press his personal views on the debated is-
> sues. To that end, I offer my own interpreta-

tions of some of the evidence and arguments employed in the white paper (107).

First, Pellegrino pointed out that the UDDA does not coincide with the proven signs of death. "Ideally," he writes, "a full definition would link the concept of life (or death) with its clinical manifestations as closely as possible," and the UDDA does not satisfy these objective findings (108). *Second*, he states: "The only indisputable signs of death are those we have known since antiquity, i.e., loss of sentience, heartbeat, and breathing; mottling and coldness of skin; muscular rigidity; and eventual putrefaction as the result of generalized autolysis of body cells" (111). The UDDA two-fold definition does not reflect death as a biological reality and is seriously flawed.

Aside from the faulty *whole-brain formulation* (endorsed by many Christian bioethicists), the "irreversible cessation of circulatory and respiratory functions" does not satisfy the UDDA's definition for organ donors. Heart and lungs harvested from one person and transplanted into another do not experience "irreversible cessation." The ventilator assists in the lungs' carbon dioxide/oxygen exchange to oxygenate the blood for registered organ donors waiting to donate. Then the beating heart circulates this blood to perfuse transplantable organs. Also, if needed, a defibrillator may be used to restart a heart, and cardiac pacing can keep the heart pumping to facilitate circulatory function in the body. The vital organs do not stop functioning, never mind reaching the point of "irreversible cessation."

The truth is that organ donors never meet the "irreversible cessation" cardiopulmonary standard. Instead, it's an educated guess based on diagnostic testing and the eagerness to *prevent* damage to a transplantable heart, lungs, and other organs due to *final stoppage* or "irreversible cessation." Since this is true, the recent ULC draft language for the revisions to the UDDA suggests using "permanent" instead of "irreversible," which has obvious problems too.

Even though declared dead under the UDDA and Dead Donor Rule (DDR), these so-called dead donors respond to anesthesia and other medications during harvest surgeries, which indicates ongoing integration between the brain, heart, and lungs to sustain life. The brain still communicates with the body via the hypothalamus, pituitary, and adrenal glands to regulate blood pressure and perform other body/brain stress responses. Contrary to popular belief, "brain dead" people with a heart and lungs healthy enough to be transplanted will not immediately stop functioning if life support is removed.

Updates to the UDDA by the ULC relate to "accepted medical standards" to determine death. According to the abstract for the 2022 "The Uniform Determination of Death Act is Being Revised" in *Neurocritical Care,* even the most fundamental question is on the table: "What are the accepted medical standards for [the] determination of death?" After nearly a half-century of harvesting organs from living donors who were declared dead under the UDDA and DDR, now it's time for an answer!

Thus far, the proposed changes by the ULC involve salvaging the UDDA, so the modifications will most likely not address its materialistic assumptions. Even if the ULC recommends updates for the "accepted medical standards" to require more sophisticated diagnostics to determine loss of brain function and bodily integration with the heart and lungs, in the end, the testing will only measure how matter/energy interact and not death as a biological fact like Pellegrino mentioned above.

We've come full circle to the original 1980 presidential commission report, *Defining Death: Medical, Legal and Ethical Issues in the Determination of Death*, which supported legislation for the 1981 UDDA "irreversible cessation of all functions of the entire brain, including the brain stem, is dead." The *whole-brain formulation*, as the neurological criterion is also known, asserts that "breathing and heartbeat are not life itself"; instead, they are "used as signs—as one window for viewing a deeper and more complex reality: a triangle of interrelated systems with the brain at its apex" (33).

According to this view, the brain is the center of life, and the heart, lungs, and bodily integration are subordinate. Death will quickly follow if someone's head is decapitated, or the brain is obliterated. However, these are not the type of people declared dead today under the UDDA neurological criterion. Instead, these people—

usually potential/registered organ donors on a ventilator—are subjectively diagnosed as having "irreversible cessation" of functions in the brain, according to "accepted medical standards" that measure how matter/energy interact.

Modern-Secular Anthropology

The prevailing story about human existence today that undergirds the UDDA is rooted in philosophical materialism. The modern story asserts we are composed solely of matter/energy derived from a big bang in the universe billions of years ago. According to this worldview, deterministic natural laws in an A+B=C fashion and complex evolutionary processes over millions of years gave rise to organic life, a variety of primates, and the human brain.

Humans are composed of six major elements from the Periodic Table: oxygen, hydrogen, nitrogen, carbon, calcium, and phosphorus, with minor amounts of sulfur, potassium, sodium, chlorine, and magnesium. All living creatures share elements from the earth. These atoms are packaged together in such a way as to form molecules (e.g., amino acids, proteins, and DNA) and cells, which create structure (anatomy) and perform functions (physiology) as the minor units of biological creatures. Humans are complex multicellular organisms with roughly 200 specialized cell types that form human anatomy and enable physiology.

A new human exists after a sperm fertilizes an egg and chromosomes unite, cells differentiate and proliferate, tissues/organs grow, bodily systems integrate, and a whole body develops. If all goes as planned during the pregnancy, the biological processes that caused life will cease sometime after the birth. At the time of death, processes causing the decay of matter/energy (that can still be measured with technology, just like living organisms) will take over, and the lifeless subatomic particles will be recycled.

What was mentioned in the last paragraph and the one above it is scientific. The first paragraph in this section, however, is a story that tries to explain how matter/energy became living organisms and human beings. Herein lies the real danger for Christians because this narrative is presented as a scientific fact when it is just another belief. The story cannot explain how matter/energy in the universe first came into existence. Neither does the hypothesis adequately demonstrate how inorganic matter/energy received the necessary properties to create organic life and, ultimately, a human being with a fully evolved cerebral cortex that seeks to understand his *or* her existence! The answer to these questions depends on the story a person accepts as authoritative, not science.

Hence, according to this view in our modern setting, the fully evolved functioning brain makes humans human and worthy of the designation "living." Yet, the Materialist has no empirical validation to support this theory other than a severed head or crushed skull. A pierced heart or collapsed lungs could satisfy this theory to define too. Therefore, the human brain cannot be at the "apex" of what it means to be a human being and living as the neurological criterion of the UDDA asserts.

The prevailing modern account of human life is fundamentally atheistic. At its best, it may only be pantheistic or deistic because it seeks to scrap the supernatural (i.e., "substances" outside this world that are different from matter/energy). These three beliefs are radically opposed to Christianity.

The Atheist denies the existence of the Creator and relies on the *assumption* of an infinite regress to explain how energy and matter came into being and made life happen. The Pantheist sees all immanence in the creation: a creator, matter/energy, and natural laws are one, and they cause life. According to the Deist worldview, the transcendence of the creator is preeminent. A divine being created matter and energy set laws into motion to govern them, and now everything occurs without divine interference.

All three of these worldviews are with us today in many disguises and they are in fundamental opposition to biblical Christianity. They are at the heart of Modern-Secular Anthropology because they try to explain the Materialist's conviction about the genesis of life mentioned in the first paragraph and its emphasis on the brain as the center of human life.

Focusing on substances obfuscates. Materialism is also called monism, and it is in opposition to dualism. Monism asserts only one substance exists, and dualism two—the former matter/energy (brain), and the latter brain and soul/spirit. According to the Dualist, the soul/spirit animates matter/energy and makes humans human and alive as brain and body beings.

Plato and Aristotle were Dualists, and so are most Christians. In simplistic terms, Plato taught the body housed the soul, and Aristotle, the soul, housed the body. Various Platonic and Aristotelian dualisms have developed in Christianity over the centuries. While a form of dualism is undoubtedly the biblical view (Holy Scripture affirms a belief in supernatural entities), placing an undue focus on substances when it comes to humans creates more problems than it solves.

The modern-day emphasis on brain/body and soul/spirit—substances—inside and outside Christendom is the product of the seventeenth-century Enlightenment. It's more helpful to set the entire substance question aside and return to the pre-Enlightenment world for answers about life, death, and our humanity. For Christians, this means returning with fresh eyes to Genesis and re-evaluating contemporary and traditional assumptions about monism and dualism that may not honor the living Creator and human life.

The Old Testament View of Humanity

I'm indebted to the Old Testament and Ancient Near East (ANE) scholar John Walton for the following insights in this section. Walton constantly reminds Christians that Holy Scripture was written: "for us, but not to us." Regarding human beings, the original author and audience were not concerned about addressing contemporary issues, like substance questions about monism and dualism. Those are our concerns, not theirs. Nevertheless, they were interested in understanding what it means to be a human created in the Creator's image.

First, Adam and Eve as archetypes. Adam and Eve are not just real people who existed at one time; their names also have significance as archetypes. Adam in Hebrew means "human," and Eve means "life." In Genesis 1:27, the man and woman are referred to as *hā' āḏām*, literally "the adam," which is not a personal name in this context. "God created man in his own image, in the image of God he created him; male and female he created them," the two archetypes of humanity.

Walton comments in *The Lost World of Adam and Eve*:

> Larger statements are being made. When the generic is used, the text is talking about human beings as a species. When the definite article is being used, the referent is an individual serving as a human representative (61).

The definite article in Hebrew is *hā'* and refers to the generic *ādām*.

Since the man was formed first, he serves as the representative archetype, but the woman is the same God-breathed dust being as the man, and she, too, is an archetype. After the tragedy in Genesis 3, "Adam named his wife Eve because she would become the mother of all the living," namely, *hā' ādām* (v. 20). Adam and Eve are transcendent/universal male and female symbols of human life.

The literal rendering of Genesis 2:7a that explains the creation of Adam as the representative of humans from Hebrew reads: "He formed the LORD God humanity dust from the ground."

English translations add "from" in front of "dust." A correct translation is "The LORD God formed humanity; dust from the ground." Humans are alive, but they are "dust," which is about mortality, not elements as defined by modern biochemistry.

The original audience would have been acquainted with the decomposition process following natural death. After a person died, the corpse was laid on a slab and went through decay. About a year later, the dust from the disintegrated body and skeletal remains were left. This is the dust the writer of Holy Scripture has in mind. It's important to note, however, that the dust returns "to the ground" from where it originally came (3:19), which can only mean the ancient Hebrews believed humans were made from the earth or material creation (cf. Ps. 139:13–15).

Second, humans with a corporate identity. Genesis 2:7b goes on to say, "and breathed into his nostrils the breath of life, and the man became a living being." The dust from the earth receives a life-giving spirit, as the Hebrew may be translated, from the Creator (cf. Job 33:4). According to

Zechariah 12:1, the Creator "forms the spirit of [human beings] (literally *hā' ādām*) within [them]." Not only does the Creator make humans from material elements, but he "forms" the spirit to animate their bodies, something supernatural other than matter/energy.

Walton comments about Zechariah 12:1, "That forming is not essentially or necessarily a material act" (71). He then cites forty-two instances in the Hebrew Bible where the verb "to form" is used in non-material ways. After the death of the body, the writer of Ecclesiastes says: "the dust returns to the ground it came from, and the spirit returns to God who gave it" (12:7).

Walton goes on to discuss the concept of establishing an identity in the ANE: "The accounts typically mention the process involved, the materials used in the creation, and the roles or functions assigned to humankind" (87). At their most fundamental level, humans are God-breathed matter/energy mortal beings with identities formed by the Creator, who serve his assigned role/function in the creation.

For the creation of Eve, Walton says Genesis 2:21 was not about the first use of anesthesia and surgery by the Creator and that more than a rib was involved in the creation of Eve. Such an interpretation reads a modern medical worldview into the text. The Hebrew word for "deep sleep" refers to a visionary state Adam experienced. Adam saw that Eve was a human like him, but she was also different because of her feminine qualities.

Thus, men and women are the same God-breathed dust beings or share an identical ontology or being, but they also have gender differences. "This is now bone of my bones and flesh of my flesh; she shall be called 'woman,' for she was taken out of man" (v. 23). Then the two will come together again for companionship, to serve as caretakers of Eden, and to procreate. "For this reason a man will leave his father and mother and be united to his wife, and they will become one flesh" (v. 24).

According to Walton, all humans share a fourfold identity as dependent God-breathed dust at their most basic level.

1. Human identity: humans are created with mortal bodies.
2. Ontological identity: humans are different

3. Gender identity: humans are male and female and will seek to procreate.
4. Relationship identity: humans are given the role of serving in the creation in a relationship with the Creator.

Surrounding this core identity is our moment-by-moment dependency on the Creator, as God-breathed dust beings.

Humans are mortal beings dependent on the creation, one another, and ultimately God. This absolute dependency must guide the Christian's approach to modern medical ethics, which needs to focus on exercising love, mercy, and compassion to fellow humans rather than prolonging life at all costs since natural death is inevitable. The human body must fulfill essential earth-bound needs to survive, reproduce, and experience wholeness. *In utero,* the fertilized egg is dependent on the mother for survival. After birth, the person requires oxygen, nutrition, security, companionship, and the involvement of others until natural death. Indeed, all humans at their core are "Dependent God-Breathed Dust."

Third, humans and their role in the creation. Genesis 2:4–24 is not a recapitulation of the sixth day of creation but a sequel to 1:26–31; Walton notes in *The Lost World of Adam and Eve* by citing several problems with the recapitulation interpretation. The passage zooms in on two specific individuals of *hā' ādām* from the *en masse* creation of humankind mentioned in Genesis 1:27–28: two individuals, Adam and Eve. Holy Scripture reveals how they were created, the sacred space they inhabited, the Creator's expectations for them, and what they are supposed to do in his creation.

Adam is to serve as the representative image bearer for Eve and *hā' ādām*. He is to depend on the Creator, follow his revealed will, and choose immortality by eating from the tree of life (see 2:16). Adam and Eve are to work together as fellow caretakers of Eden in their roles as a male and female, fill the creation with fellow image bearers to extend Eden's borders, and rule the earth as the Creator's visible vice-regents.

According to Walton, Eden was an area set apart from the rest of the creation as a sacred space. In the ANE context, this calls to mind temple complexes, beautiful gardens, and domesticated animals. Ziggurats in ancient Mesopotamia served as stairs for the gods to descend to the earth. Next to the ziggurat was a temple for the deity to reside. This was Eden minus the ziggurat and temple, for the Creator already dwelt in Adam and Eve's midst (3:8). John picks up on this imagery in Revelation 21 in his description of the renewed creation or worldwide Eden. The Creator appointed Adam and Eve as priestly caretakers of his sacred space.

As we all know, God's creation project was derailed because Adam ate from the forbidden tree. Genesis 2:16, the "LORD God commanded the man, 'You are free to eat from any tree in the garden'" but forbade only one, the "tree of the knowledge of good and evil" (v. 17). The result of eating from this tree was misguided dependency, alienation from God, and death. The Creator banished the rebellious duo from Eden. "After he drove the man out," the writer of Genesis says, "he placed on the east side of the Garden of Eden cherubim and a flaming sword flashing back and forth to guard the way to the tree of life" (3:24).

Now the ability to become immortal was forfeited, and death reigned over them and the entire human race. "Therefore," writes Paul in Romans, "just as sin entered the world through one man, and death through sin, and in this way, death came to all men because all sinned" (5:12). Nevertheless, even though Adam chose the tree of knowledge and death/mortality, the obligations of the Creator to obey his revealed will still stand for *hā' ādām* — humankind is still accountable to God.

The Wages of Sin is Death

Cain's murder of his flesh and blood brother Abel puts the heinousness of Adam's first sin on display. Cain had a total disregard for the Creator of life, human life, and his faithful brother's life. After the horrific event, "the LORD said to Cain, 'Where is your brother Abel?' 'I don't know,' he replied. 'Am I my brother's keeper?' The LORD said, 'What have you done? Listen! Your brother's blood cries out to me from the ground" (Gen. 4:9–10). The Creator banishes Cain even further away from Eden, and his main concern is not the total disregard he had for Abel's life; it's about preserving and prolonging his own (vv. 13, 14).

The subsequent total disregard for human life is mentioned in Genesis 4 in connection with Cain's great-great-grandson Lamech. He boasts about murdering a male youth and mocks the Creator of life. Lamech said:

> I have killed a man for wounding me, a young man for injuring me. If Cain is avenged seven times, then Lamech seventy-seven times (vv. 23–24).

Previously, the Creator said to Cain, "if anyone kills Cain, he will suffer vengeance seven times over" (v. 15).

Lamech thinks he is untouchable because God showed mercy to Cain. Walton comments in *The NIV Application Commentary: Genesis*:

> The text has moved from unrepentant Cain to defiant Lamech. Violence is glorified, and the mark of Cain no longer stands as a stigma of exile but as a badge of honor that brings protection equivalent to invulnerability. The human situation is degenerating (278).

"Now the earth was corrupt in God's sight and was full of violence" (6:8).

The Creator finally brings judgment but not

before an act of saving grace to Noah (v. 11).

> God said to Noah, "I am going to put an end to all people, for the earth is filled with violence because of them. I am surely going to destroy both them and the earth" (v. 13).

Noah and his family are spared. After dealing with the human brutality, the Creator establishes the death penalty for those who commit acts of murder: "Whoever sheds the blood of man, by man shall his blood be shed; for in the image of God has God made man" (9:6).

As the story of Holy Scripture and world history unfolds, there is still a disregard for human life right up to the present day. Cain is another archetype in contrast to Adam, Eve, Abel, and Noah, who represent repentance, restoration, and redemption (cf., 4:24; Luke 3:38). Cain is the archetype of the self-centered murderer, who defies the revealed will of God, and takes the Creator of life for granted.

John warns Christians:

> Do not be like Cain, who belonged to the evil one and murdered his brother. And why did he murder him? Because his own actions

were evil and his brother's were righteous. Do not be surprised, my brothers, if the world hates you. We know that we have passed from death to life, because we love our brothers. Anyone who does not love remains in death. Anyone who hates his brother is a murderer, and you know that no murderer has eternal life in him (1 John 3:12–15).

The line of Cain is with us today.

What Cain represents is revealed in modern-day assumptions about life and death that devalue human life and defend acts of murder. The spirit of Cain is reflected in laws like the UDDA and those that safeguard on-demand abortion. It is the Creator revealed in Holy Scripture who gives life to a fertilized egg in the womb, and it's the Creator who takes his spirit back when he chooses.

Of course, the Creator is omnipotent or all-powerful, and even the murderous acts of humans fit into his eternal plan in some way. Nevertheless, the human obligation to do the Creator's revealed will according to scientific facts is compulsory. Holy Scripture is clear: "You shall not murder" (Exod. 20:13). Actively ending the lives of fellow God-breathed dust with biological signs of life is murder, even if these humans are cells in a womb or declared "brain dead" with a beating heart on a ventilator.

Prolonging life at all costs is not up to us either since this is the Creator's prerogative and natural death is inevitable. Our goal is to show our fellow mortals love, mercy, and compassion (Luke 10:30–38). Withdrawing a ventilator or withholding aggressive life-prolonging treatments may be the most loving, merciful, and compassionate thing to do for a person diagnosed as "brain dead" or a baby born with congenital abnormalities. When to pursue, withdraw, or withhold these types of treatments are complex choices beyond the scope of this book. Nevertheless, Christians need to remember that God is in control and his timing is always impeccable (Eccles. 3:1–2).

Contrary to the story underlying "Modern-Secular Anthropology," all humans possess a particular type of life endowed by the Creator of life revealed in Holy Scripture; namely, his life-giving spirit that animates matter/energy/cells to create human anatomy, and to set into motion physiological processes. Adam and Eve are the archetypes of human life, and as God-breathed dust beings different from other creatures, they gave birth to fellow humans with XX (female) and XY (male) chromosomes. As the Creator's vice-regents, men and women are to care for the creation according to God's revealed will, which means caring for one another as mutually "Dependent God-Breathed Dust" in relationship to the Creator as bearers of his image in the world.

2

Unique Image-Bearers
with a Purpose

All humans receive life from God, share a fourfold identity, and depend on the creation and Creator for survival. At our most basic level, this is what it means to be a human being created in the image of God. Is there more, however, to God's image in humans? According to Christian theologians, the answer is yes, and they are right. However, the way some of them define the image of God is in terms of attributes or faculties, which is wrong.

For example, the *Evangelical Dictionary of Theology* describes the image of God this way:

> Evangelical expositors of the biblical revelation find the created image of God to exist formally in human personality (moral responsibility and intelligence) and materially in his knowledge of God and his will for humanity. ...The biblical view is that humanity is made to know God as well as obey him (593).

Aside from appealing to Aristotle's theory of causation to define the Hebrew concept of the image of God, the implication is only those with moral, intellectual, or volitional abilities reveal the Creator of life. Not to mention, Aristotle was a pagan whose ideas were shaped by a Greek worldview that put idols and human reason at the center, not the God of Holy Scripture. The article on the image of God offered by the *Evangelical Dictionary of Theology* is not biblical.

All humans are created in God's image regardless of rational knowledge, moral obedience, or volitional ability. Walton comments in *Ancient Near Eastern Thought and the Old Testament*:

> Across the ancient world, the image of God did the work of God on the earth. In the Israelite context as portrayed in the Hebrew Bi-

ble, people are in the image of God in that they embody his qualities and do his work. They are symbols of his presence and act on his behalf as his representatives (212).

The ancient pagan religions, like those during Aristotle's day, believed the idols they created represented a god, and their work earned the deities' favor. Israelite religion turned this around. God creates his image bearers to declare his existence, and he fulfills his purposes in the creation through them.

Notice the biblical view is more about what the Creator does and not what human beings do. Neither is the image of God dependent on knowledge of the Creator or his will or in human personality, as referenced in the *Evangelical Dictionary of Theology*. Holy Scripture teaches that all people, individually and corporately, "are in the image of God in that they embody his qualities and do his work," are "symbols of his presence," and "act on his behalf as his representatives."

Humans declare the Creator's existence because they are "symbols of his presence." According to the introductory article for the *Dictionary of Biblical Imagery*:

> A *symbol* is an image that stands for some-thing in addition to its literal meaning. …symbolism emerges as a shared language in a culture (xiv).

An *image* is literal and concrete. Humans are *de facto* created in the image of God—they have ontology or being. As *symbols*, humans reveal the existence of the Creator by their presence in the creation.

Walton goes on to say in the *Lost World of Adam and Eve,* "it is essential to affirm that all people are in the image of God, regardless of their age, their physical ability or inability, their moral behavior, their ethnic identity, or their gender" (42–43). Theologian Herman Bavinck, *Reformed Dogmatics,* agrees with Walton: "Nothing in a human being is excluded from the image of God" (2:555).

God's spirit unites with the genetic matter in a sperm and egg union at conception to create a human. At this point, the living God's image is present in a new person that is mortal, given gender (XX or XY chromosomes) and is related to the Creator and creation as a dependent being. Beyond this core identity, this person displays the Creator's image like no one else in the world, and he *or* she serves the Creator's specific purpose in the creation.

Jesus: The Second Adam

After Adam rebelled, human beings did not lose the image of God, but it was distorted. Sin, at its core, is a radical distrust of the Creator's revealed will and devotion to misguided dependency. The incarnate life, death, resurrection, and ascension of Jesus in history, the Second Adam, addressed Adam's rebellion.

> For this reason he had to be made like them, fully human in every way, in order that he might become a merciful and faithful high priest in service to God, and that he might make atonement for the sins of the people. ...For we do not have a high priest who is unable to empathize with our weaknesses, but we have one who has been tempted in every way, just as we are—yet he did not sin (Heb. 2:17; 4:15).

Jesus was made like the first Adam, "fully human in every way," but "he did not sin." Indeed, as the Second Adam, he was an image bearer of God as a human being who not only paid the price for sin as an unblemished sacrifice (atonement), but he started a reversal of its effects in the creation as the only sinless high priest, serving as king *and* priest after the order of Melchizedek (5:10).

Considering what we know about *in-utero* development today, thinking about the Son of God becoming a human is astonishing. After Jesus was supernaturally conceived in Mary's womb, God's breath of life united with genetic matter to create a symbol of the Creator's presence. Jesus was a mortal human related to the Creator and the creation as a dependent person. Beyond these essential human characteristics, Jesus also had a unique identity and was appointed to serve the Creator's specific purpose in the creation. According to Holy Scripture, this staggering historical fact about Jesus is just as indisputable as the *in-utero* beginning of our individual lives.

Jesus has a unique identity. For Jesus, the human being, this identity did not come from his divinity or experiences after he was born. Jesus' identity preexisted in the "mind" of the Father,

Son, and Holy Spirit—the Trinity. The mortal human, Jesus, is distinct from the eternal Son of God, as the *Westminster Confession of Faith* summarizing the Chalcedonian Creed states:

> The Son of God, the second person in the Trinity, being very and eternal God, of one substance and equal with the Father, did, when the fullness of time was come, take upon Him man's nature, with all the essential properties and common infirmities thereof, yet without sin; being conceived by the power of the Holy Ghost, in the womb of the Virgin Mary, of her substance. So that two whole, perfect, and distinct natures, the Godhead and the manhood, were inseparably joined together in one person, without conversion, composition, or confusion. Which person is very God, and very man, yet one Christ, the only Mediator between God and man (8:2).

The wording "two whole, perfect, and distinct natures…without conversion, composition, or confusion" avoids conflating the human and divine identities of Jesus. Yet these "distinct natures, the Godhead and the manhood, were inseparably joined together in one person."

Since Adam's sin and death infected the entire human race, the sinless Son of God needed to become a human being to cure the infection (see Rom. 5). Philip Edgcumbe Hughes, in *The True Image: The Origin and Destiny of Man in Christ,* explains:

> It was by means of the virgin birth that the Son of God took our human nature to himself. ...The incarnation...relates back to and interprets the original unique act of creation ...which had been dragged down by the [sin] of the first Adam. ...[I]t was necessary for Jesus Christ, the last Adam, to enter the world like the first Adam, innocent, God-centered, unstained by sin, and unburdened by guilt. ...It was the birth of Jesus from a virgin mother, our fellow human being, that preserved the vital connectedness with our human nature (261).

The "innocent, God-centered, unstained by sin, and unburdened by guilt" eternal Son of God was united to the temporal human Jesus, "the son of Adam, the son of God" (Luke 3:38). Jesus became a part of *hā' āḏām* as the Second Adam. Beyond this, he was the person Jesus who had a preexistent and unique human identity before the creation.

While we will never know the full extent of our unique selves, these were not obscure facts about Jesus. Mary knew her unborn son's preexistent identity because the angel Gabriel revealed it to her:

> You will conceive and give birth to a son, and you are to call him Jesus. He will be great and will be called the Son of the Most High. The Lord God will give him the throne of his father David, and he will reign over Jacob's descendants forever; his kingdom will never end (Luke 1:31–33).

As the passage describes, the human being developing in her womb will be named Jesus. He is the divine Son of God. He will assume the throne of his ancestor, king David, reign over Israel or "the children of the promise" (Rom. 9:8), and his earthly kingdom will never end.

Holy Scripture affirms a view of identity referred to as "essentialism." This view contradicts the philosopher John Locke's *tabula rosa* or "blank slate theory," which says identity is formed solely by sensory experience and consciousness after birth—the prevailing view today. According to psychologist Dr. Daniel Robinson, *The Mind*, essentialism is the commonsense view of one's identity. He explains:

> Common-sense understanding is that one must have a mind for experiences to be had; that even though one's body and brain are in constant flux, there is an "essential" or "substantial" self that endures through all such (merely) physical transformations …One retains one's defining and "essential" nature even as one matures (288).

The "essential" or "substantial" self is the "mind" or the human spirit formed by God in a biblical worldview (Zech. 12:1). It was the God-breathed spirit that ultimately gave Jesus his unique identity, not his conscious experiences after birth—the same is true for everyone (cf., Heb. 2:17). This essential self was in the eternal "mind" of the triune Creator, and it was united to genetic matter in Mary's womb during the reign of Augustus Caesar (63 BC–AD 14).

The Son of God became incarnate as a unique image bearer of the Creator of life, "the man Christ Jesus" (1 Tim. 2:5):

> The Word became flesh and made his dwelling among us. We have seen his glory, the glory of the One and Only, who came from the Father, full of grace and truth (John 1:14).

The Son of God united with God-breathed dust. Jesus, the male, was dependent on Mary *in utero*. After his birth, he required oxygen, nutrition, security, companionship, and the involvement of other people to grow and develop. Therefore, as a fellow image bearer, Jesus was able "to sympathize with our weaknesses" (Heb. 4:15).

Jesus also experienced human misery and mortality. He suffered and died a natural death. On the cross, "Jesus called out with a loud voice, 'Father, into your hands I commit my spirit.' When he had said this, he breathed his last'" (Luke 23:46). The human spirit formed by God returned to him (Eccles. 12:7), and Jesus' corpse was laid on a stone slab in Joseph of Arimathea's tomb.

The Second Adam was fully human with a unique identity, and it was always in the "mind" of the triune Creator to do something more than create an Adamic race after the likeness of the first Adam. Recall Hughes's comment above, Jesus "relates back to and interprets the original unique act of creation." The Creator's purpose was never aimed only at Adam and a creation project; it always had in the background a redemptive program that required the incarnation of the Second Adam and restoration of the creation (see Eph. 1:3–14).

Jesus has a unique purpose. The Second Adam was "the Lamb who was slain from the creation of the world," and this preordained purpose testifies to the image of God in the Second Adam as well (Rev. 13:8). In the early years after Jesus' crucifixion (atonement for sin), the disciples "raised their voices together in prayer to God. 'Sovereign Lord,' they said

> Herod and Pontius Pilate met together with the Gentiles and the people of Israel in this city to conspire against your holy servant Jesus, whom you anointed. They did what your power and will had decided beforehand should happen (Acts 4:27–28).

Those are astonishing words! Two individuals and people groups, who despised each other, collaborated to execute Jesus. Even more remarkable, above all the human hostility, the entire historic event was what the Father, Son, and Holy Spirit's "power and will had decided beforehand should happen." Puzzling, but this is the God of Holy Scripture.

All faithful Christians believe in a triune Creator—Father, Son, and Holy Spirit— who is self-existent, all-knowing, all-powerful, unchangeable, and perfect. God is not limited by time and space. He is infinite and eternal. God is independent from his creation; he is not a part of it. God is all-knowing; he cannot gain new knowledge. God is all-powerful; he cannot be controlled. God is unchangeable; he cannot change. Since God is perfect, his ultimate purpose in creation cannot be modified, confounded, or thwarted. Plan A will not fail, so there is no plan B. Everything that occurs is "in accordance with his pleasure and will" (Eph. 1:5).

Jesus achieved victory over Adam's sin for others, which is pure GRACE (God's Riches At Christ's Expense).

> Since the children have flesh and blood, he too shared in their humanity so that by his death he might break the power of him who holds the power of death—that is, the devil— and free those who all their lives were held in slavery by their fear of death. For surely it is not angels he helps, but Abraham's descendants. For this reason he had to be made like them, fully human in every way, in order that he might become a merciful and faithful high

priest in service to God, and that he might make atonement for the sins of the people. Because he himself suffered when he was tempted, he is able to help those who are being tempted (Heb. 2:14–18).

Only another human being could deliver fellow image-bearers out of their Adamic predicament. So, the second person of the Trinity agreed to become Jesus. The Second Adam accomplished what the first Adam failed to do as a priestly caretaker and vice-regent of Eden. Jesus became the leader of a renewed humanity by making atonement for Adam's sin as the preordained Lamb who was slaughtered. As the last high priest of the Aaronic priesthood, he offered himself as the final old covenant sacrifice to provide access to the most holy place (see Heb. 8–10).

The temple system in Jerusalem was terminated after Jesus died on the cross (Matt. 27:51; Mark 15:37; Luke 23:45). Jesus prophesied about the temple's destruction, which took place once and for all in AD 70 (Luke 19:41–44). At present, the Holy Spirit is building a new temple by uniting image-bearers of the Creator of life to the

Second Adam through a new non-*in-utero* birth (John 3:3).

> Consequently, you are no longer foreigners and strangers, but fellow citizens with God's people and also members of his household, built on the foundation of the apostles and prophets, with Christ Jesus himself as the chief cornerstone. In him the whole building is joined together and rises to become a holy temple in the Lord. And in him you too are being built together to become a dwelling in which God lives by his Spirit (Eph. 2:19–22).

"The children of the promise," whether they are Jews or Gentiles, are "Abraham's seed" and "Jacob's descendants," who are "born from above" individually to "become a holy temple in the Lord" corporately as the Second Adam's visible Body in the world, the Church.

Writing about the event with the Samaritan woman at Jacob's Well, John quotes Jesus as saying:

> "Woman," Jesus replied, "believe me, a time is coming when you will worship the Father neither on this mountain nor in Jerusalem. You Samaritans worship what you do not know; we worship what we do know, for salvation is from the Jews. Yet a time is coming

and has now come when the true worshipers will worship the Father in the Spirit and in truth, for they are the kind of worshipers the Father seeks. God is spirit, and his worshipers must worship in the Spirit and in truth" (John 4:21–24).

In John 2, Jesus said to the Jews who reviled him: "Destroy this temple, and I will raise it again in three days" (2:19). John explained, "the temple he had spoken of was his body. After he was raised from the dead, his disciples recalled what he had said" (vv. 21–22).

Jesus, the Son of God, is "Immanuel (which means 'God with us')" (Matt. 1:18). This was Eden's temple in Genesis 3:8, and it's the temple of Revelation 21. Locality no longer matters because the Second Adam rose from the dead, and "the true worshipers will worship the Father in the Spirit and in truth" throughout the world to renew the earth as "a chosen people, a royal priesthood, a holy nation" (1 Peter 2:9). Habakkuk prophesied long ago, saying, "the earth will be filled with the knowledge of the glory of the LORD as the waters cover the sea" (2:14).

Paul explains the eternal purpose of the Sovereign Lord for his priestly caretakers and vice-regents in these last days before the Second Adam's return:

> For those God foreknew he also predestined to be conformed to the image of his Son, that he might be the firstborn among many brothers and sisters. And those he predestined, he also called; those he called, he also justified; those he justified, he also glorified (Rom. 8:29–30).

The Christian's goal in life is glorification, which means being "conformed to the image of [God's] Son" by striving to live a love-filled life, dying a faithful natural death, and hoping for a bodily resurrection. This is nothing less than the Christian's undying passion for renewing the creation according to the Creator's revealed will in Holy Scripture and the facts of science.

In his contribution to *The Lost World of Adam and Eve*, "Excursus on Paul's Use of Adam," New Testament scholar NT Wright expands on Jesus' role as the Second Adam in the larger context of the Creator's purpose for the creation. After developing the background for Paul's Jewish worldview, Wright zooms in on Romans. "The great climax of Romans 1–8 is the renewal of all creation," he writes, "in Romans 8:17–26, where Jesus as Messiah, with reference to Psalm 2, is given as his inheritance the uttermost parts of the world."

After the Second Adam's resurrection and before his ascension, Matthew quotes Jesus as saying:

> All authority in heaven and on earth has been given to me. Therefore go and make disciples of all nations, baptizing them in the name of the Father and of the Son and of the Holy Spirit, and teaching them to obey everything I have commanded you. And surely I am with you always, to the very end of the age (Matt. 28:18–20).

There is now a resurrected human image-bearer ruling over the creation, seated at the living Creator's right hand. The Son of God and glorified Second Adam exercises his gracious rule in the creation at present through the Creator's chosen "vessels of mercy," Christians, by his Spirit (Rom. 9:23). The Second Adam accomplished what the first Adam failed to do by living a sinless life and by his death on the cross for "the sin of the world" (John 1:19). The Second

Adam satisfied the Creator's punishment for what Adam did. Now the glorified Second Adam waits for the triune Creator's command to return to the earth in person.

Romans 5 is at the heart of the Adam and Second Adam parallels and contrasts. Wright, in his discussion, focuses on verses 17 and 21:

> For if, by the trespass of the one man, death reigned through that one man, how much more will those who receive God's abundant provision of grace and of the gift of righteousness reign in life through the one man, Jesus Christ! …so that, just as sin reigned in death, so also grace might reign through righteousness to bring eternal life through Jesus Christ our Lord.

He writes:

> Adam's sin meant not only that he died but that he lost the "reign" over the world. God's creation was supposed to function through human stewardship, and instead it now produces thorns and thistles. …Paul's Adam-theology is also his kingdom theology …Grace reigns "through righteousness" to the life of the age to come. God sets people right in order that through them he will set the world right. Justification by faith is God putting people right in advance, in order that

through them God will put the world right (174).

Christians are justified by grace through faith in the Second Adam. They trust the Creator's revealed will and strive after a properly aligned dependency on the Creator and creation. They pray for God's kingdom to come, and they hunger and thirst after righteousness to usher it into the world. When Christians live like this, they bring heaven and earth together. They are putting the Creator's creation project back on track as redeemed image-bearers of God in his recreation project.

According to Wright, this is the Christian commitment to live out the image of the Creator of life in the creation. "The image is a *vocation*, a calling," or a purpose. "It is the call to be *an angled mirror*, reflecting God's wise order into the world and reflecting the praises of all creation back to the Creator" (175). The first Adam was supposed to do this as a bringer of life, but he chose the curse of death. Why? A more glorious eternal purpose orchestrated by the Father, Son, and Holy Spirit was in the background—redemption.

The Second Adam accepted death and restored life through his glorified resurrection body as the forerunner of a renewed Adamic race (cf. 1 Cor. 15:20). Redeemed image bearers will strive to be bringers of life. They seek to live out their unique identities to fulfill the Creator's redemptive purpose at present as "vessels of mercy," even while they look forward in hope to the Second Adam's return and to an immortal resurrection body like his. Wright concludes with this warning: "if you choose to worship and serve the creation rather than the Creator, you will merely reflect death back to death, and will share that death yourself" (178).

Living as God's Redeemed Image-Bearers

What does all of this have to do with *When Christians Say, "I Believe Life Starts at Conception?"* Everything!

First, the way the image of God is defined in many Christian traditions can potentially devalue human life. Not only are these formulations unbiblical, but they couldn't anticipate the advances in medicine and ethical dilemmas we face today. People lacking mental capacity and volition, like unresponsive organ donors on a ventilator and unborn babies in a womb, still bear the image of God. If biological signs of life are present, a unique image bearer of the Creator of life with a purpose is alive. According to the revealed will of God in Holy Scripture, these vulnerable people are not to be murdered and exploited by fellow humans.

Second, all humans are God-breathed dust, share a fourfold identity, and are dependent beings. God's breath of life was united with genetic matter to create a unique image bearer to serve his purpose in the world. All of us are unlike other creatures, were assigned a gender, are mortals, and are related to the Creator and the creation as dependent beings. There was never a time, nor will there ever be, when we did not depend on others and the material world.

We relied on our mothers *in utero*. After birth, we require oxygen, nutrition, security, companionship, and the involvement of other people to grow and develop. The biblical view of the image of God is more about what the Creator is doing with the biological material he brings to life, not what humans do intellectually, morally, or volitionally. We mutually depend on one another for ongoing survival, and Christians should champion this dependency by being dependent on the Creator and his revealed will.

Third, everyone has an identity that is unique to her- or himself that testifies to God's image in the creation. As noted above, we share a corporate identity as members of humanity. Still, there is a specific preexistent uniqueness the Creator has conferred on each of us that no one else shares. While experiences in life help us understand who we are, our gifts and our callings, God's breath of life make each of us uniquely us. Life is a journey of self-discovery that becomes truly authentic after being born again by the Holy Spirit into the family of the Second Adam. No one enters the world as a blank slate, and the unique identity the Creator conferred on each person fits into his creation project and eternal purpose in some way.

Fourth, all of us serve the Creator's purpose as bearers of his image in the drama of redemption. Christians no longer follow the defiant ways of the first Adam and murderous Cain; they are in union with the resurrected and glorified Second Adam as "vessels of mercy." Now they seek to trust the Creator's revealed will in Holy Scripture, strive to exercise a proper dependency on the creation and Creator, and advocate for God-breathed dust.

Jesus was once asked by a teacher of the Law: "Of all the commandments, which is the most important?"

> "The most important one," answered Jesus, "is this: 'Hear, O Israel: The Lord our God, the Lord is one. Love the Lord your God with all your heart and with all your soul and with all your mind and with all your strength.' The second is this: 'Love your neighbor as yourself.' There is no commandment greater than these" (Mark 12:29–31).

Jesus quoted Deuteronomy 6:4–5 and Leviticus 19:18 in his response, namely, the revealed will of the Creator. These exhortations are the spirit behind this book's interpretation of the Sixth Commandment: "You shall not murder" (Exod. 20:13).

Aborting an unborn baby and cutting organs out of a "brain dead" donor with a beating heart are hateful acts toward the Creator of life. Before the Sixth Commandment, there was another prohibition against actively ending human life for self-serving/exploitative reasons in Genesis 9:6. This explains why abortion and harvesting organs from unresponsive people with biological signs of life are so tragic: "for in the image of God has God made mankind." According to the revealed will of God Jesus quoted, unborn babies and unresponsive people on ventilators are *always* to be cherished, protected, and loved because they possess a particular type of life—a human life that bears the Creator of life's image in his creation as God-breathed dust.

3

Dualism and Its Dangers

Before we consider "Dualism and Its Dangers," it will be helpful to briefly explore the rise of materialism in psychology. Recall that this view is also referred to as monism and opposes dualism. The idea of materialism has been around since pre-Socratic philosophers, but it is a recent development in the philosophy of mind. In the mid-seventeenth century, the atheistic philosopher Thomas Hobbes suggested human beings were biological machines. In 1747, the French physician Julien Offray de la Mettrie took the next step and published an entire book called *Man a Machine* (accessed www.gutenberg.org).

In this book, La Mettrie asserted that humans "are at bottom only animals and machines." He continues:

> The human body is a machine which winds up its own springs. It is the living image of perpetual movement. Nourishment keeps up the movement which fever excites. Without food the soul pines away, goes mad, and dies exhausted.

Explaining his use of the word "soul," or the human spirit formed by God in a Christian worldview (Zech. 12:1), La Mettrie said: "soul is...an empty word."

Without scientific evidence and in one fell swoop, La Mettrie jettisoned dualism, opted for monism, and laid the foundation for materialism in its various mutations for modern studies of the mind. According to La Mettrie, "the soul is but...a material and sensible part of the brain, which can be regarded...as the mainspring of the whole machine." Elsewhere he writes, "This principle exists and has its seat in the brain at the origin of the nerves, by which it exercises its control over the rest of the body."

The next significant move in the philosophy

of mind came with the neuroanatomist and physiologist Franz Josef Gall and his theory of phrenology. Gall believed that distinct brain regions were responsible for thoughts, emotions, personality, and behavior. According to Gall, mental states result from processes in the brain, like steam rising from a pot of boiling water (epiphenomena). Thus, the real work of thinking, feeling, behaving, and even consciousness occurs exclusively in the brain's defined regions. Gall came to his conclusions by studying the bumps on people's heads.

Today, "bumpology," the pejorative term for phrenology, is more detailed and comprehensive. Psychiatrist Jeffrey Schwartz, in *The Mind & The Brain*, explains the goals of phrenology and compares them with the objectives of modern neuroscience:

> This belief has dominated studies of mind-brain relations since the early nineteenth century, when phrenologists attempted to correlate the various knobs and bumps on the skull with one or another facet of personality or mental ability. Today, of course, those correlations are a bit more precise, as scientists, going beyond the phrenologist's conclusion that

thirty-seven mental faculties are represented on the surface of the skull, do their mapping with brain imaging technologies such as positron emission tomography (PET) and functional magnetic resonance imaging (fMRI), which pinpoint which brain neighborhoods are active during any given mental activity (23).

Areas in the brain are assigned a variety of operations in correlation with matter/energy activity detected by modern-day imaging studies that are related to the impairment/loss/gain of a mental, sensory, or motor function caused by a substance, injury, or a disease in a region of the brain. For the definition of mind, or soul/spirit, materialism under its various formulations has become the *indisputable dogma* of modern medicine today.

According to neuropsychiatrists, the front of the head, or prefrontal cortex, is responsible for higher-level thinking, working memory, and personality. The front sides of the head, or temporal lobes, are associated with hearing, interpreting language, and emotional responses. The middle sides of the head, or parietal lobes, possess various sensory processes, temperature regulation, and spatial awareness. The back of the head, or occipital lobe, is involved in processing visual stimuli. The cerebellum, or the "little brain," affects movement, balance, and posture.

Several vital structures are deep within the cerebral cortex or midbrain. The basal ganglia are responsible for initiating movement. The thalamus and hypothalamus regulate essential functions between the brain and body. The limbic system includes two critical substructures, the hippocampus and amygdala: the first regulates emotions and the second long-term memories. The reticular formation is involved with sleep and wake cycles. Finally, the brainstem regulates vital body functions to sustain life.

The brain has billions of neurons and neuronal interconnections at the cellular level. Besides these neurons in the brain, billions are also in the body's spinal cord and systemic nervous system. Each part is interconnected and integrated with the body. Even after a couple of centuries of research, neuroscientists have only begun to scratch the surface of the complex interplay between neurons, dendrites, synapses, and neurotransmitters—matter and energy. Never mind providing scientific explanations to explain how neurochemical activity in the brain becomes a dream, thought, idea, or belief. While commonsense points us in the direction of a master integrator for matter/energy, such as a spirit/soul/mind, the Materialist declares emphatically, "No!"

For people committed to monism, there are some vexing problems. Since we're all made of identical matter and have the same neuronal cause/effect processes, why don't we think, feel, believe, and behave the same way? What about our unique personalities and proclivities? What about people with literally half a brain that live high-functioning lives? How does matter and energy become consciousness, thinking, feeling, believing, and personhood?

What fills the gap between neurochemical functions at the level of dendrites, synapses, and neurotransmitters to cause those events we usually associate with the mind/soul/spirit? There is a close relationship between the events, that's for sure. We know that ingesting or injecting a material substance can alter mental states, but the reverse is true: mental activity can change brain and body processes. Psychologist Dr. Daniel Robinson comments in his lecture, "The Explanatory Gap," *Consciousness and Its Implications*: "Not every relationship is a causal relationship, nor does correlation imply causality," when it comes to the brain and mind (15).

Besides all of what was mentioned above, what about the hunch that guided these gifted neuropsychiatrists with their distinctive personalities, who felt called to unlock the mysteries of the brain? What inspired these brilliant women and men to engage in this journey of discovery? Was it merely useless byproducts of neurological activity from the brain that floated above their heads? People committed to monism deny the reality of their unique drives, feelings, beliefs, and aha moments that influence their actions!

Carl Yung, *Modern Man in Search of a Soul*, gives six other examples of these types of mental events on page 187:

1. Emotions we can't suppress
2. Moods we find difficult to change
3. Dreams we are powerless to stop
4. Obsessive thoughts that cause impulses
5. Memory lapses we experience

6. Imagination that can transport us

Along with inspiration, these *objective events experienced subjectively* indicate another reality beyond matter/energy, cause/effect, and even conscious experience.

What about the question of human existence people share from every time and place? A *stream of subconsciousness awareness* reflected in universal or transcendent symbols as archetypes written in stone, scrolls, and books. The genesis of human life in Christianity is understood by looking to the fully formed body/brain of Adam (human) and Eve (life) with a Creator and breath of life (spirit) in the background.

The Modern-Secular Anthropology account is radically different from the Christian narrative, but it is still a non-scientific story about the genesis of human life. *Miraculously* subatomic particles came into existence, *mysteriously* somatic cells came to life, and *hypothetically* through random and then finely tuned evolutionary processes over millions of years humans with a fully evolved brain came into being.

Writing in the early twentieth century, Jung

wrote in the same book mentioned above:

> It was universally believed in the Middle Ages as well as in the Greco-Roman world that the soul is a substance. Indeed, mankind as a whole has held this belief from its earliest beginnings, and it was left for the second half of the nineteenth century to develop a "psychology without the soul." Under the influence of scientific materialism, everything that could not be seen with the eyes or touched with the hands was held in doubt; such things were even laughed at because of their supposed affinity with metaphysics. Nothing was considered "scientific" or admitted to be true unless it could be perceived by the senses or traced back to physical causes (177).

He goes on to say: "a metaphysics of the mind was supplanted in the nineteenth century by a metaphysics of matter," and he was correct (178). Monism is just as scientifically bankrupt as dualism because both make *assumptions* about reality, which is what the study of metaphysics is all about.

Two Bodily States and One Spiritual Identity

For Christians, one would expect a commitment to some form of dualism, but this is not always the case. For example, New Testament scholar Joel Green, in "Three Exegetical Forays into the Body-Soul Discussion," *Criswell Theological Review*, says: "N.T. Wright observes, 'We have been buying our mental furniture for so long in Plato's factory that we have come to take for granted a basic ontological contrast between "spirit" in the sense of something immaterial and "matter" in the sense of something material, solid, physical.'" While Wright is concerned about Platonic influences in Christianity and with what he calls the New Testament doctrine of "after afterlife" (see *The Resurrection of the Son of God*), Green is trying to eliminate dualism from Christianity by affirming monism (see *Body, Soul, and Human Life*).

Aside from many passages in Holy Scripture that indicate the existence of supernatural entities like the Holy Spirit, a God-breathed human spirit, angels, and "ghosts," Jesus' non-animated body/brain was laid in a tomb. However, the human spirit formed by the Creator was still alive with the repentant criminal "in paradise" (cf. Luke 23:43). It is also a well-documented fact that the ancient Jews believed the human-spirit hovered around the corpse immediately after death. Whatever view a biblical scholar takes about paradise, the apparent conclusion from Holy Scripture and history is Jesus continued to live on as an ontological human spirit.

Luke writes in 23:46: "Jesus called out with a loud voice, 'Father, into your hands I commit my spirit.' When he had said this, he breathed his last." A plain reading of this text asserts two simultaneous events: (1) Jesus committed his spirit to his Father, and (2) he breathed a final breath and died.

According to the passage cited above, the human spirit of Jesus returned to the Creator after he stopped breathing, and he joined the crucified criminal who defended him on the cross "in paradise." Joseph of Arimathea lowered Jesus' corpse from the cross and laid it in his tomb. If there are only "material, solid, physical" things, then there was no ongoing existence for Jesus, the person, with the Father and repentant criminal.

Of course, the historic resurrection accounts in the Old and New Testaments also support dualism. The prophets Elijah and Elisha were used by the Creator of life to resurrect two dead boys (1 Kings 17:17–23; 2 Kings 4:19–37). In the New Testament, Jesus resurrected the synagogue ruler's girl (Mark 5:38–42), the widow of Nain's son (Luke 7:11–15), and Lazarus (John 11:38–44). Then there were the resurrections of Dorcas by Peter (Acts 9:36–42) and Eutychus by Paul (20:9–10). The account recorded in 1 Kings 17:21–22 explains these types of resurrections the best: Elijah "cried out to the Lord, 'Lord my God, let this boy's life return to him' …the boy's life returned to him, and he lived."

There are also accounts of people in Holy Scripture who died or were taken but still have their same unique identities. The inspired writers mention Samuel in the Old Testament (1 Sam. 28) and Moses and Elijah in the New (Matt. 17:3–8), along with the cloud of witnesses in Hebrews 11 – 12:1 and the martyrs in John's revelation (Rev. 6:9–11). Before launching into his teaching on the glorified resurrection body in 1 Corinthians 15, Paul provides a taxonomy of "bodies" in verses 35–41: animals, birds, fish, "heavenly bodies," "earthly bodies," sun, moon, and stars. Why not human spirit "bodies," since there are also angelic bodies?

Paul also mentioned being caught up in heaven, "Whether it was in the body or out of the body I do not know—God knows" (2 Cor. 12:2). This experience was more than a vision like John's (Rev. 9:17), Peter's trance (Acts 10:10), or even Paul's nightly vision of the Macedonian (Acts 16:9). Paul had an experience where he thought his spirit was separate from his still biologically alive body. While Paul willingly admits ignorance before God about this disembodied state, he sees it as valid. He just accepted that it happened and did not give answers to our numerous questions about it.

Nevertheless, Paul still had much to say about the human body in its present and future states. The Greek word for body is *soma*, and it's best to use this term when Paul speaks about the body. Paul does not have in mind a body as distinct from a soul as Plato or Aristotle taught. Instead, Genesis 2:7 and Jewish anthropology forms his thinking. Paul means a body-spirit union as a "living being" or "living soul" when he uses *soma*.

According to Siegfried Wibbing's article in

the *New International Dictionary of New Testament Theology*, three themes underlie Paul's use of *soma* (1:234):

1. There is a somatic or bodily existence. The *soma* (even at conception) testifies to a unique person's presence, a union of body-spirit.
2. The *soma* is the essential person. One's identity in the spirit is one with the body.
3. The present *soma* and the resurrected *soma* are the same person. The difference is a state of existence.

A person's God-breathed spirit, in Paul's understanding, Wibbing writes, "is thinkable only in a body...an earthly or 'physical body' and a 'spiritual body.'"

According to Paul, those in union by faith with the Second Adam are a *soma psychikon* and one day will become a *soma pneumatikon* to introduce two more Greek terms. Paul writes in 1 Corinthians 15:44–47:

it is sown a natural body, it is raised a spiritual body. If there is a natural body, there is also a spiritual body. So it is written: 'The first man Adam became a living being'; the last Adam, a life-giving spirit. The spiritual did not come first, but the natural, and after that the spiritual.

The emphasis is not on substance (natural/physical and spiritual) but on states of existence, first as a natural/physical body (*soma psychikon*) and later as a spiritual body (*soma pneumatikon*).

Paul says the different states are like being "unclothed" at one time and then "clothed" at another (see 2 Cor. 4–5). It's the same person who was once naked (a natural/physical body or *soma psychikon*) and is now dressed (a spiritual body or *soma pneumatikon*). The *soma psychikon* represents a present body as an image-bearer of the living God. The *soma pneumatikon* is the Christian's future body in the likeness of Jesus' resurrected body—a glorified image-bearer of the Creator of life (see Rom. 8:29–30).

What about those who are not Christians? Will they have a resurrected body? The short answer is yes, but it will not be a *soma pneumatikon* like the Second Adam; it will be some type of *soma psychikon* prepared for everlasting death. As Wright said, people who live in this world choosing to "reflect death back to death" will "share that death." As noted in chapter one, "the obligations of the Creator still stand for *hā' ādām*—humankind is still accountable to God." Those who persist in rebellion against the Creator of life will receive his just punishment.

One of the most challenging doctrines in Holy Scripture taught by Paul is found in Romans 9. In this chapter, he says God has made "vessels of mercy" and "vessels of wrath" (vv. 22–23). Both are image bearers of the triune Creator that serve his eternal purpose, which is the person's ultimate end in the creation. The former reveals God's attribute of mercy, and the latter justice—both are "symbols of his presence," as Walton said earlier.

Once again, Paul does not satisfy our inquiries and rebukes those who question God's eternal will (vv. 19–21). People who reject Jesus will experience a bodily resurrection to be judged "for the things done while in the body, whether good or bad. ...those who have done what is good will rise to live, and those who have done what is evil will rise to be condemned" (2 Cor. 5:10; John 5:29). The "good" is trusting the Creator's revealed will as it is revealed in Holy Scripture and striving after a properly aligned dependency on the Creator and creation.

The Creator's revealed will is clear: he does not want "anyone to perish, but everyone to come to repentance" (2 Peter 3:9). According to Holy Scripture, people are not prevented from humbling themselves and acknowledging dependency on the God of Holy Scripture. All who seek after life (immortality) and ask the Second Adam for it as a *soma psychikon* will receive it (Luke 11:10–13). No one is barred access to the Second Adam. The Son of God became a *soma psychikon* to redeem people, and if humans reject him, the triune Creator is not to blame.

God created Adam's body from material creation, breathed life into it, and Adam became a *soma psychikon*. While living in this body, Adam rebelled against God's command. He was banished from Eden and lost access to the tree of life. The Second Adam came into the world as a *soma psychikon*. He obeyed the Creator of life and paid the penalty for Adam's rebellion. The Second Adam put on the garb of resurrection glory as the first *soma pneumatikon* to give life to all who desire to rise from the dead with him spiritually at present and bodily at his second coming.

The continuity between both bodies is God's breath of life, not the present *psyche* or the future *pneuma*. Wibbing comments: "The body, in the sense of the 'I,' the 'person,' will survive death through the creative act of God" (1:236). The "creative act" refers to the life-giving spirit God unites to matter/energy or genetic material at conception to create a *soma psychikon*. This unique image-bearer of the Creator of life serves his eternal purpose as a member of *hā' ādām* in the creation, and he *or* she does so ultimately as a "vessel of mercy" or "vessel of wrath."

Some Dangers Associated with Dualism
Paul's "letters contain some things that are hard to understand," as Peter once said (2 Peter 3:16). Especially since he testifies to his own out-of-body experience, other types of "bodies," and a glorified resurrection body at the second coming of Jesus. The historical resurrections mentioned in the Old and New Testaments create further perplexity. Not to mention the affirmation of historical saints reappearing as mentioned in Holy

Scripture, such as Samuel, Moses, Elijah, the cloud of witnesses, and martyrs.

Jesus' death and three-day presence as a human spirit with the repentant criminal's spirit "in paradise" adds further confusion. Paul focuses on the bodily resurrection because this is the Christian's hope, which is not a disembodied state "In the Sweet By and By"—that's why things are complicated. Wright's comment above is aimed more at this issue and not the monism Green is injecting into Christianity. Nevertheless, substance dualism has some real dangers, and we will briefly consider two major categories: theological and practical.

The first problems are theological. Some Christians emphasize the doctrine of salvation, a disembodied state after death, spirit/soul as more important than the body/brain (matter/energy), a bodily resurrection, and the renewal of the material creation at Jesus' second coming. CS Lewis once commented:

> God never meant man to be a purely spiritual creature. That is why He uses material things like bread and wine to put the new life into us. We may think this rather crude and un-

spiritual. God does not: He invented eating. He likes matter. He invented it.

Christians who indulge, abuse, or neglect the body tend to adopt views that value the soul/spirit over the "flesh," body, or *soma*. These extremes dishonor the Creator who made the material body. Closely connected with what was mentioned above is a focus on "saving souls" and the hope of becoming a disembodied soul/spirit after death.

Although these views are prevalent among many Christians, they are not biblical. Since these theological issues are beyond the scope of this book, I'll direct the reader to Wright's excellent treatment of them in *Surprised by Hope*. These theological issues were important to mention, however, because they lay a foundation for a distorted Christian worldview and, therefore, the Christian's understanding of the beginning and end of life as a human being.

The second problems are practical. When emphasizing the soul as a substance or as having greater value than the body, a Dualist may view unresponsive people on ventilators with a beating heart as dead. Since the Uniform Determination of Death Act (UDDA) was made law in 1981, this position has prevailed among Christians. It is reflected in the acceptance of the *whole-brain formulation* of death. According to this view, the part (soul/spirit/personhood) that matters is no longer present with the biologically *alive* body, which is an idea developed from the evolution of various forms of substance dualism in Western philosophy, not Holy Scripture.

Recall how some of the philosophers at Athens dismissed Paul when he mentioned the *soma pneumatikon* of Jesus (Acts 17:22–32). The elites referred to Paul as a bird picking seeds out of manure. Those who mocked him saw the ideal state as a soul separated from the body, but Paul taught the opposite. His focus was on a resurrected body, or a *soma* as defined above, with life — a biological life like Jesus' resurrected body that ate food (cf. Luke 24:41–43) — not on a disembodied, ethereal state.

I've been at the bedside of people with objective signs of life on ventilators diagnosed as legally dead under the *whole-brain formulation* of the UDDA. I've heard Christians say, "Our son has died and gone on to be with the Lord," and decide to donate organs based on medical advice rooted in monism and the Dualist theological problems mentioned above. There are also Christians who receive organs from people in these conditions and do so after the counsel of leaders in the Church.

If biological signs of life are present in the *soma psychikon*, a union of spirit/soul/mind and brain/body is still present. The God-breathed spirit is still with the body even though the person on a ventilator is diagnosed as being "brain dead." She *or* he still bears the image of God as a unique person with a purpose. The representative of the Creator of life is to be blessed by the love, mercy, and compassion of fellow God-breathed dust, even if it's for a few minutes after the withdrawal of a ventilator until a final breath is expired and the heart stops beating.

When Christians Say, "I Believe Life Starts at Conception" and call abortion murder but believe it is acceptable to harvest organs from "brain-dead" people, they're inconsistent. Why would a non-responsive person with a beating heart on a ventilator be viewed as dead but non-developed cells in a womb dependent on a mother as living? According to Holy Scripture, both possess the Creator's breath of life, and both bear the Creator's image.

While Christians may hold to a consistent dualism for the unborn baby, for the brain-dead organ donor, their dualism collapses into monism. Namely, right into the story that says supernatural entities don't exist. Jesus' three-day separation as a human spirit from his corpse is a prescientific idea of the ancients. The miraculous events of the incarnation and resurrection are superstitious myths concocted by the deluded but hopeful followers of Jesus. As for eternal life here and now: "Well, that's just the empty by-product of the limbic system/neocortex due to the release of dopamine into synapses—a mechanism of the brain to help gullible people cope with death."

If Christians believe life starts at conception, it doesn't end until human beings breathe their last breath, and the God-breathed spirit returns to the Creator of life.

4

"Life Unworthy of Life"

A wicked policy in Germany was *Lebensunwertes Leben*, a phrase translated into English as "life unworthy of life." This 1920 doctrine permitted euthanasia for image-bearers of the Creator of life with congenital abnormalities, developmental problems, and mental impairment. The ideas undergirding the *Lebensunwertes Leben* eventually gave rise to the horrors of Nazism in Germany and an attempt to exterminate the Jews. It then fueled the totalitarian obsession of Hitler to attain world domination where only those deemed worthy had a right to life.

Robert Jay Lifton explains in his 1986 *New York Times Magazine* article, "German Doctors and the Final Solution":

> Nazi "euthanasia," in fact, provides a key to an understanding of genocide as inclusive murder of the victim group in order to "cure" one's own. Since the disease one seeks to eliminate is ultimately death itself, the curative process can be endless. That murderous cure must be combated, interrupted, prevented everywhere.

Approximately 6 million Jews, 5,000 children born with genetic deficits, and 200,000 people with neurocognitive problems met their demise under the *Lebensunwertes Leben* policy. A program directed and supervised by medical doctors in Germany.

Sadly, some of the *Lebensunwertes Leben* ideas were also supported in America in the early twentieth century. In 1916, eugenics supporter and founder of Planned Parenthood, Margaret Sanger, established the nation's first "birth control clinic." In 1927 the United States Supreme Court ruled to permit compulsory sterilization for people deemed "unfit." *Lebensunwertes Leben* did not die out after World War II either, and policies that devalue life in the United States (US) continue.

More than 63 million abortions have occurred since 1971. Eighty percent of unborn babies diagnosed with Down Syndrome, anencephaly, spina bifida, and other congenital disabilities are aborted. These babies who are never born are said to have conditions of "life incompatible with life." On the other end of the spectrum, fully developed people with objective signs of life are declared dead under the Uniform Determination of Death Act (UDDA) and referred to as "cadavers" or corpses. This represents 90 percent of the organ donors that are said to meet the Dead Donor Rule (DDR) in the US.

The *Lebensunwertes Leben* impetus is the same in America, especially for those judged dead with transplantable organs; end the lives of those less fortunate, because those deemed more privileged are worth more. All of this may seem shocking but consider, *The Permission to Destroy Life Unworthy of Life* (translated to English from German) in comparison with the "Report of the Ad Hoc Committee of the Harvard Medical School to Examine the Definition of Brain Death." The former was written in 1920 and laid the groundwork for the Nazi policy of *Le-*

bensunwertes Leben. The latter was published in 1968 and served as the impetus to redefine death in the US to allow organ procurement from "brain-dead" donors with objective signs of life.

Reputable experts in their respective fields wrote both documents. These elites discuss physicians' legal role in determining the line between life and death, the futility of care for those in altered mental states, the economic burden these people cause to society, and how others deemed more worthy can benefit from them.

"The Permission to Destroy Life Unworthy of Life," writes Lifton, revealed that "a policy of killing was compassionate and consistent with medical ethics." He says the authors "pointed to situations where doctors were obliged to destroy life—interrupting a pregnancy to save the mother, for example." Further, the writers "claim that various forms of psychiatric disturbance, brain damage and retardation indicated that the patients were already 'mentally dead.'" The authors "characterized these people as 'human ballast' and 'empty shells of human beings.'" According to the writers, Lifton continues, ending these people's lives "is not to be equated with other types of killing [and it is] an allowable, useful act."

"Report of the Ad Hoc Committee of the Harvard Medical School to Examine the Definition of Brain Death" states:

> Our primary purpose is to define irreversible coma as a new criterion for death. There are two reasons why there is need for a definition: (1) Improvements in resuscitative and supportive measures have led to increased efforts to save those who are desperately injured. Sometimes these efforts have only partial success so that the result is an individual whose heart continues to beat but whose brain is irreversibly damaged. The burden is great on patients who suffer permanent loss of intellect, on their families, on the hospitals, and on those in need of hospital beds already occupied by these comatose patients. (2) Obsolete criteria for the definition of death can lead to controversy in obtaining organs for transplantation.

The committee desires to redefine death for those in a "coma" judged by a physician to be in a "mentally dead" condition that is "irreversible" but "whose heart continues to beat." These dehumanized people are nothing more than "cadavers," heart-beating corpses dependent on life support, "human ballasts," and "empty shells of human beings." They are a burden to themselves due to their "loss of intellect, on their families, on the hospitals, and on those in need of hospital beds."

Nevertheless, they are valuable to society since they possess perfused organs that can be transplanted into those deemed more fortunate. If an "irreversible coma [is] a new criterion for death," we can legally murder these people by cutting out their healthy hearts, lungs, livers, kidneys, and other organs. Harvesting organs from these people "is not to be equated with other types of killing [and it is] an allowable, useful act." The Chairman of the Harvard Ad Hoc Committee, Dr. Beecher, was blunt and candid in a 1967 lecture: "Can society afford to discard the tissues and organs of the hopelessly unconscious patient when they could be used to restore the otherwise hopelessly ill but salvageable individual?"

The similarities between the two documents are striking, along with the cold and inhuman attitudes that undergird them. Equally remarkable is the proliferation of propaganda associated with both ideologies.

Americans have wondered how so many Germans could've accepted the horrific acts committed in Nazi Germany. Bruce L. Shelley, *Church History in Plain Language*, makes the following suggestion as to why:

> Christianity has been displaced by an ideology that creates a mass party for some totalitarian government. The party, however, is always led by a dictator or a small but dedicated ruling elite, who commands a political police force. By the use of sophisticated, psychological methods the rulers are able to direct the minds and emotions of the people against the "enemies" of the regime. Propaganda and control of the media, along with the regulation of the economy, are aimed at producing a new type of people utterly lacking any hunger for personal freedoms (420).

First, an ideological agenda is advanced by a dedicated elitist class with financial, academic, and political power seeking to control society. *Second*, clever methods are devised to persuade and guide the thinking and feelings of the public by controlling the media, regulating the economy, and developing a story for people to believe. As Shelley notes, the propaganda is "aimed at producing a new type of people utterly lacking any hunger for personal freedoms." *Third*, those in the minority opposing the ideology are marked as miscreants in opposition to what is "best for society"; namely, the ideological agenda, or, yes, story of the elitist class in power.

UDDA Propaganda in the US Exposed

An instance of "life unworthy of life" propaganda in the US was seen in the media's confusion about the death of Anne Heche and the public's responses to it. On August 11, 2022, Heche was declared dead under the neurological criterion of the UDDA in California. The actress desired to be an organ donor. Although legally dead, Heche was kept alive for three more days to harvest her organs.

Newspapers reported she died on August 11 and 14. *The Washington Post* published an internet article, "Why the media declared Anne Heche dead twice," and some of the responses to the publication underscore the ideology associated with the Nazi *Lebensunwertes Leben* and the power of UDDA propaganda.

Adam Bernstein, the obituary editor, did not

recognize brain death as a clear indicator of death. "It's black and white. There's no gray area here. If you're on life support, you're still alive," Bernstein was quoted as saying in "Why the media declared Anne Heche dead twice." The public's reactions to Bernstein's statement reveal the successful propagandizing of the public by the pro-UDDA elites:

> If WP doesn't acknowledge brain death as death, that's anti-scientific and potentially damaging for the public, possibly leading to instances of relatives struggling to accept that their loved ones are dead. ...One root of the problem lies in the words we use. The term "life support" is imprecise. While "life support" machinery may indeed support life (provided that the patient is alive), what they do is to support and uphold bodily processes like circulation of blood, gas exchange in the lungs, and filtration of waste products and so on. ...These processes are necessary for life, but they can also occur in a dead body, or even in tissue removed from the body. If needed, these vital organs may be transferred, through organ donation, from one body to another ...If you're brain dead (provided the diagnosis is made correctly, by competent physicians) you're dead, and there is no more life to support. If your body may show some semblance of life, like the color of skin, o[r]

chest expanding on inflation, that is the results of machines and drugs working on the body. ...Time of death is when brain death occurs, or more pragmatically when it is diagnosed.

If you're brain dead, you're dead. That's what being dead is. Every organ or tissue of your body may be damaged, repaired, removed or even replaced. But your brain may not be removed or replaced — because it's you.

Brain death is death. Hard stop. After that, you are just a bunch of organs available to be harvested.

A brain dead person is basically a beating heart cadaver.

The people who made these comments were unaware of the ongoing controversy surrounding brain death and harvesting organs from these types of donors.

As recently as May 14, 2021, Dr. Alan Shewmon, a retired Professor of Neurology and Pediatrics at the University of California, and 107 experts in medicine, bioethics, philosophy, and law recommended public transparency when it comes to the brain-death criterion of the UDDA. Shewmon authored "Statement in Support of

Revising the Uniform Determination of Death Act and in Opposition to a Proposed Revision" in *The Journal of Medicine and Philosophy: A Forum for Bioethics and Philosophy of Medicine*. According to the article abstract:

> Finally, objections to a neurologic criterion of death are not based only on religious belief or ignorance. People have a right to not have a concept of death that experts vigorously debate imposed upon them against their judgment and conscience; any revision of the UDDA should therefore contain an opt-out clause for those who accept only a circulatory -respiratory criterion.

The way Heche was declared dead is not a settled matter, which is why the Uniform Law Commission (ULC) is seeking to update the UDDA.

In 2018, Harvard Medical School hosted "Defining Death: Organ Transplantation and the Fifty-Year Legacy of the Harvard Report on Brain Death." According to the experts at the conference, the brain-death criterion of the UDDA is a legal fiction, and the DDR does not represent the fact of death (i.e., the absence of biological signs of life) when based on the UDDA. In a speech, "The Dead Donor Rule as Policy Indoctrination," David Rodriguez-Arias said:

> policymaking becomes indoctrination whenever public opinions and preferences are intentionally manipulated in ways that destroy or prevent citizens' independent judgment and rational deliberation. ...The history of death determination in the context of organ donation can be described as an indoctrinating attempt to settle a moral controversy.

Before 1981, the dehumanizing comments made about Anne Heche and the authoritative statements by the public referring to brain death as death would have only been made by a small, dedicated class. Most people, physicians included, in the US during that time would've viewed someone in a coma with a beating heart on a ventilator as severely incapacitated but not dead. The 1968 article by Beecher was the first move to change this narrative in the US. The policymakers and propagandists of the UDDA have succeeded in brainwashing and controlling large portions of the public, as the comments attached to *The Washington Post* article show.

The first pundit cited reflects this indoctrination profoundly. "If WP doesn't acknowledge brain death as death, that's anti-scientific and potentially damaging for the public, possibly leading to instances of relatives struggling to accept that their loved ones are dead." The moral controversy is settled for this writer. Those who question Heche's death are "anti-scientific," and they will harm family members and the public. The brainwashed person boldly proclaims, *The Washington Post* needs to correct its article!

Recall Dr. Pellegrino's statement from chapter one: "Ideally, a full definition would link the concept of life (or death) with its clinical manifestations as closely as possible" (108). A beating heart, breathing lungs, and functioning body that interacts with the brain, even with mechanical assistance and drugs, indicate ongoing life for those committed to pursuing science. Dead bodies don't do anything; they're dead!

It's important to emphasize the point above, especially since Christians distinguish between *resurrection* and *resuscitation*. People die on ventilators and life-sustaining medications every day.

Hundreds also die with implantable defibrillators and pacemakers. Medical technology and drugs may support vital functions in a living body, but they cannot restore living processes in a biologically dead body. The difference is between *resurrection* (a supernatural event like animating a sperm-egg union in a womb) and *resuscitation* (a natural event that requires the ongoing animation of the body by a God-breathed spirit).

Death is a disintegration of vital organ systems, tissues, and cells after the heart and lungs stop. Once the standard of irreversible cessation *in truth* is met, the person's life cannot be restored, and vital organs suffer immediately from oxygen deprivation. At the time of natural death, a systemic disruption of anatomical and physiological processes occurs in the whole body that medical technology cannot reverse, not even in a single vital organ that has crossed the biological line from life to death.

In a 2009 edition of *Medicine, Health Care, and Philosophy*, "Brain death, states of impaired consciousness, and physician-assisted death for end-of-life organ donation and transplantation," the researchers concluded that surgically removing the organs from donors meeting the *whole-brain formulation* of death was the actual cause of death for these donors. They add that this "prevailing practice is being performed with no public disclosure ignoring the need for a broad ethical, medical, and legal debate in society," and this publication was more than a decade ago (421).

Doctor Heidi Klessig and I co-authored *Harvesting Organs and Cherishing Life: What Christians Need to Know About Organ Donation and Procurement* to raise awareness about these living donors murdered by the removal of their organs. The recent deliberations of the ULC to update the UDDA provides evidence for the integrity of the 2009 article mentioned above, and our 2021 book.

Shewmon suggested, "Just as cigarette ads are required to contain a footnote warning of health risks, ads promoting organ donation should contain a footnote along these lines: 'Warning: It remains controversial whether you will actually be dead at the time of the removal of your organs.'" Doctors Franklin Miller and

Robert Truog, in *Death, Dying, and Organ Transplantation: Reconstructing Medical Ethics at the End of Life*, write: "As a way of approaching the ideal goal of honest engagement with the legitimacy of vital organ donation from still-living patients we advocate making these legal fictions transparent by acknowledging that death in the eyes of the law is not the same as death in fact according to a biological definition" (153).

Statements based on law do not always represent the facts of science. For example, the Health Resources & Services Administration (HRSA) dogmatically states: "Brain death is death and it is irreversible." According to Truog and Miller, "patients have been legally diagnosed as dead according to the standard criteria, only to begin breathing…in the interval between the diagnosis of brain death and the onset of organ procurement." Shewmon has documented 175 cases of "brain dead" people who lived after the declaration of death, some for more than twenty years. Many have even recovered after a diagnosis of "irreversible cessation of all functions of the entire brain, including the brain stem."

As the responses to *The Washington Post* article indicate and the present-day organ donor registry shows, the "life unworthy of life" propaganda advanced by the US's financial, academic, and political elites has been effective. Clever methods were devised to persuade and guide the thinking and feelings of the public, like connecting Valentine's Day with National Donor Day.

Licensed drivers are also aware of the posters at the Department of Motor Vehicle (DMV) sites around the country encouraging organ donation. A seemingly innocuous ploy to motivate giving "the gift of life," aimed at invincibly minded teens and young adults with healthy organs. A split-second *uninformed consent* is given to a DMV window attendant, a decision that sets *mandatory* and *irrevocable policies* in motion after a major automobile accident under the Uniform Anatomical Gift Act (UAGA).

The ploys are successful. According to Organdonor.gov, in "2021, 169 million people in the US have registered as donors," far exceeding the number of organ donors needed. Presently, only 106,036 people are on the organ transplant registry. The population in the US for 2021 was 332 million. More than 50 percent of Americans were registered as organ donors that year. Roughly 3,458,697 people died in 2021, so statistically, 1,729,349 registered organ donors died. Nevertheless, the United Network for Organ Sharing (UNOS) reported, "13,861 people became deceased organ donors nationwide in 2021."

Why is this number so low? The reason is 1,715,488 registered donors crossed the line from life to death, so their dead vital organs could not be transplanted. Organdonor.gov explains: "only 3 in 1,000 people die in a way that allows for deceased organ donation." That "way that allows" is the "life unworthy of life" policy of the UDDA that defines people as dead who are still alive. One that kept Heche alive for three days after a legal declaration of death to harvest her body parts, as Bernstein correctly reported.

Like the smoke that billowed from the chimneys in Auschwitz, a successfully propagandized public trusts the persuasive ideology of the elites doing what is "best for society." These people are manipulated and socially engineered by the authoritarian regime to become desensitized to reality and to embrace with zeal the morals/ethics manufactured for them based on the "facts of science"; namely, the pro-UDDA story, another narrative like Hitler's at odds with commonsense and Christianity.

Christians need to rise like Dietrich Bonhoeffer and oppose the "life unworthy of life" doctrine in the US. Brain death is not death, which is why the 2008 Presidential Council examined the issue and recommended using "total brain failure" and even wondered if "total" accurately represented the condition. The Council declared:

> It may be helpful to emphasize that the word "total" in the phrase, "total brain failure," refers to the fact that the brain injury has reached the endpoint of a process of self-perpetuating destruction of neural tissue. In any event, whether or not the word "total" is justified, the patient diagnosed with total brain failure is in a condition of profound incapacity, diagnostically distinct from all other cases of severe injury. Whether this state of profound incapacity warrants the determination of death remains a matter of debate, with advocates of the neurological standard arguing it does, which critics maintain it does not (38).

The UDDA neurological criterion is not a settled matter, especially for Christians who believe life starts at conception. The brain does not develop until five weeks into the pregnancy, so based on this fact alone, brain death cannot equal death. For Christians, it is best to see "brain-dead" people as Jesus portrayed the victim in the parable of the Good Samaritan, who was described as "half dead" and in need of the love, mercy, and compassion of a neighbor (Luke 10:30–38). These people deserve the kindness, empathy, and benevolence of fellow dependent God-breathed dust, not the exploitative tactics of greedy harvest mongers.

One of the significant effects of the first Adam's sin through the line of Cain is seen "as inclusive murder of the victim group in order to 'cure' one's own," as Lifton mentioned above. In our case, the victims are organ donors subjectively diagnosed with "irreversible cessation" of the whole brain with a beating heart on a ventilator. They are declared dead based on a legal fiction at odds with God's Law and scientific facts, with no public transparency.

Nothing displays humanity's inhumanity

more than the will to euthanize vulnerable people by surgically removing their healthy organs and transplanting them into another person deemed more worthy to live.

> Brain death is death. Hard stop. After that, you are just a bunch of organs available to be harvested.

Like the propagandized *Washington Post* commenter cited above, Hitler's brainwashed followers made similar statements, which is why Lifton stated in his article:

> Since the disease one seeks to eliminate is ultimately death itself, the curative process can be endless. That murderous cure must be combated, interrupted, prevented everywhere.

Postscript

Here is an example of how I connect the historical narrative of Holy Scripture to my present life story each day. After I get up in the morning, I remember Genesis 3:19: "for dust you are and to dust you will return." I recall that I'm God-breathed dust dependent on the Creator and creation for ongoing survival and that I have a unique identity and purpose as a symbol of God's presence in the world.

I remember my life is more about what the Creator has done by creating me than what I do. I also remind myself that God's ultimate purpose for me is to be a "vessel of mercy." To this end, I'm to act as his representative in the creation. I've been redeemed for this purpose. I'm to use my unique personality, gifts, and calling to be a pro-life advocate for the vulnerable and a minister of compassion so that heaven will come in some measure to the earth.

Then I sit, pray, and meditate. Before reading the morning selection in *The Psalter*, I open with, "Glory be to the Father, the Son, and the Holy Ghost, as it was in the beginning, is now..." At this point, I remind myself that roughly 2,022 years have elapsed since the Son of God was incarnated as a human being; I recall the day of the month, the day according to the Fourth Commandment, and the liturgical season the Church is presently celebrating. I then conclude with, "ever shall be world without end. Amen."

The *Gloria Patri* doxology has succinct theology reaching back to the eternal Trinity, to the future "world without end," and to a present "now," my life today. It transcends time and space, sets the context for the Christian's present story, and invites me into the lived historical, spiritual, and psychological experiences recorded in *The Psalter*.

Equally crucial in *Gloria Patri* is its focus on the "world" or creation. Many of the psalms also speak about the creation and, more specifically, about the Creator and the vice-regency of humankind over it. Much of this was mentioned in chapters one and two, so I will not write about it here. The renewal of the creation as "a chosen people, a royal priesthood, a holy nation" is crucial to living out the Christian story in the present (see 1 Peter 2:9–12).

Not to mention the grid through which past, present, and future fits—the same "as it was in the beginning" with the Trinity. The doxology and psalms have everything to do with the Creator's eternal purpose in the everlasting or renewed creation (see Eph. 1:3–14), which has nothing to do with the spirit/soul leaving the body behind to enter an otherworldly existence, but everything to do with a bodily resurrection in the renewed creation at Jesus' second coming. I talked about the importance of this perspective in chapter three. ***Christians are to cherish human life even in its most reduced states because this unique person is still alive in the creation, bears God's image, and serves the eternal purpose of the Creator.***

After *The Psalter* selection, I rehearse the Ten Commandments as affirmations, which is the spirit of the Law. I rejoice that I have an exclusive and sincere love for the Creator, characterized by a desire to glorify his name in the world by living out his revealed will for life (1–3). I'll skip to the Sixth Commandment affirmation: "to cherish life." I commented on this at length throughout the book. This commandment has special significance because of how the Creator formed my spirit, my experiences in life, and his ultimate purpose to create me to be a "vessel of mercy." My heartfelt goal is to apply this commandment by striving to love the Creator and my neighbor while living in a world of darkness that does not desire to do his will, devalues human life, and exploits the vulnerable for self-centered reasons.

Let's oppose the "life unworthy of life" doctrine in the US! Don't fear those in power. Confront them boldly, but do so with meekness, wisdom, love, prayer, and sincerity. Show compassion to those who had an abortion or donated/received an organ from a person declared dead under the Uniform Determination of Death Act (UDDA). Be consistent in your pro-life convictions since modern medicine routinely develops treatments and products from human body parts derived from immoral and unethical procedures (a resource to help navigate these issues is www.respectforhumanlife.com).

Don't be a registered organ donor because if you're declared dead by US law, you will be euthanized by having your organs removed — you may also be aware of what is happening during the organ harvest surgery! Registering as an organ donor will also serve as your consent to active euthanasia if you're diagnosed as legally dead under the UDDA. Stipulate in writing and explain to family members your refusal to accept the UDDA as a valid definition of death.

It is always necessary to remove a ventilator and to wait for the heart and lungs to stop functioning before a declaration of death can be made. Of course, this means no vital organs to transplant from this truly dead person who has reached the standard of irreversible cessation of the heart, lungs, and brain, but there is nothing wrong with donating a body after biological death.

After the ventilator is withdrawn, it's essential to allow the administration of medications to ease agitation and breathing. The purpose of the drugs is not to cause death, but it is an act of compassion that will reduce suffering. In God's providence, the person on may live on—most do—for several minutes, hours, weeks, months, and years without a ventilator. Several have even recovered. The extra time is a blessing from the Creator of life to show love, mercy, and compassion to another human being, not a burden to be endured.

Above all, remember in this present story of life: "If we live, we live for the Lord; and if we die, we die for the Lord. So, whether we live or die, we belong to the Lord" (Rom. 14:8).